Journal of Health Politics, Policy and Law

Volume 47, Number 2, April 2022

Published by Duke University Press

Board of Editors

Contents

Special Issue
Racism, Health, and Politics

Special Issue Editors: Jamila Michener and Alana M. W. LeBrón

Racism, Health, and Politics: Advancing Interdisciplinary Knowledge

Jamila Michener
Cornell University

Alana M. W. LeBrón
University of California, Irvine

Racism and health predominated political agendas across (and beyond) the United States in the spring of 2020. The simultaneous calamities of the COVID-19 pandemic and the murder of George Floyd underscored the urgency and interconnectedness of racism and health. Even as COVID-19 was disproportionately devastating Black, Latina/o/x/e, Pacific Islander, and Native communities, people across the United States were participating in massive, historic protests against racialized state violence (Barber 2020, 2021; Buchanan, Bui, and Patel 2020; Escobar et al. 2021; Lopez, Hart, and Katz 2021; Putnam, Chenoweth, and Pressman 2020). In this context, racism was declared a public health crisis, states and cities discussed policy solutions, institutions of all stripes had moments of "racial reckoning," and partisan politics became even more divided over whether and how to address racism (Andrews 2021; Blake 2021; Vestal 2020; Yearby et al. 2020).

Notwithstanding the urgency of these events, the intersecting forces of racism, health, and politics were central features of American life long before the spring of 2020. Throughout US history, political institutions, markets, and social structures have developed, maintained, embodied, and enforced practices of racial categorization and differentiation (Bailey, Feldman, and Bassett 2021; Bateman, Katznelson, and Lapinski 2018; King and Smith 2005; Omi and Winant 2014; Rothstein 2017; Williams 2003). This has been particularly evident in the realm of health, where policies, politics, laws, and ideas have produced racial inequities (Bailey and Moon 2020; Hahn, Truman, and Williams 2018; Hardeman, Hardeman-Jones, and

Journal of Health Politics, Policy and Law, Vol. 47, No. 2, April 2022
DOI 10.1215/03616878-9517149

Medina 2021; Mateo and Williams 2021; Michener 2020; Phelan and Link 2015; Pirtle 2020; Wailoo 2014; Washington 2006; Williams and Collins 2001; Williams, Lawrence, and Davis 2019). Systems of racial stratification shape whether you live in a neighborhood that will promote your health, have access to resources to sustain your health, have daily experiences that will threaten your health or make you vulnerable to illnesses that will weaken your health, and they influence the political processes that can be activated to protect your health (Carter et al. 2017; LaVeist 1992; Mateo and Williams 2021; Wailoo 2014; Wallerstein 1992; Williams and Collins 2001; Williams and Mohammed 2013; Zelner et al. 2021).

Though many of these social processes are now widely recognized as drivers of health and health inequities (IOM 2003; Smedley, Stith, and Nelson 2003), they have proven resistant to change (Lurie 2005; Zimmerman and Anderson 2019). Despite advances in knowledge about racial health inequities (Kneipp et al. 2018), progress toward effective solutions has been slow and sometimes inverted. Politics is a key reason for the chasm between what we know about health and racism on the one hand, and what we have (and have not) changed on the other. This dynamic is vividly illustrated by the COVID-19 pandemic. In response to the emergence of the novel coronavirus, researchers developed abundant scientific knowledge about vaccines, masking, other mitigation efforts, social determinants of health, and structural determinants of racial health inequities. Such knowledge has proven crucial for identifying strategies to fight the pandemic and related inequities that have disparately burdened low-income communities and communities of color (Akee and Reber 2021; Hooper, Nápoles, and Pérez-Stable 2020; Ong et al. 2020). Yet the reach and influence of science was constrained by politics. Politics emerged in partisan divisions over policy responses to COVID-19, ideological rifts over the role of the government, the politicization of data collection, controversies over the interpretation and veracity of scientific research, and much more (Clinton et al. 2021; Gadarian, Goodman, and Pepinsky 2021; Michener 2021). Nearly all these political battles have implications for racial (in)equity. In this way, COVID-19 highlights integral connections between racism, health, and politics (Bailey and Moon 2020; Hooijer and King 2021).

Such connections are evident in many policy domains. For example, scholars who study immigration have identified critical linkages between politics, processes of racialization, and health (Kline 2019; LeBrón et al. 2018a; LeBrón et al. 2018b; LeBrón et al. 2019; Lopez 2019; Cruz Nichols,

LeBrón, and Pedraza 2018a, 2018b; Novak, Geronimus, and Martinez-Cardoso 2017; Pedraza, Cruz Nichols, and LeBrón 2017; Young, Beltrán-Sánchez, and Wallace 2020). Similarly, a small but burgeoning literature on Medicaid policy has amplified the tripartite significance of racism, health, and politics in that arena (Franklin 2017; Grogan and Park 2017; Lanford and Quadagno 2016, 2021; Leitner, Hehman, and Snowden 2018; Michener 2018, 2020, 2021; Snowden and Graaf 2019).

These examples only scratch the surface. Close examination of many policy areas underscores the imperative and intersecting importance of racism, health, and politics. Nevertheless, popular and scholarly discussions of these topics tend to be siloed. Substantive engagement with the health implications of racism is often divorced from larger questions about politics and policy. At the same time, scholarship centered on politics and policy is often disconnected from the realities of structural racism in health—the ways it is perpetuated through public health and health care systems, experienced by racially marginalized populations, mitigated through policy channels, and more.

Recognizing these lacunae, this special issue of the *Journal of Health Politics, Policy and Law* assembles a leading group of multidisciplinary scholars. Bringing together researchers who might otherwise operate in separate spheres, the special issue augments and integrates scholarship that advances knowledge of health, racism, and politics across disciplines and fields of study.

Conceptual Clarification

To situate and contextualize the topical focus of this special issue, we offer some conceptual clarification. The complexities, confusion, and even convolution endemic to discourse around race and racism make this an important first step. Health and politics are also variably comprehended and worth elucidating. Though the articles in this special issue proffer (either explicitly or implicitly) their own distinct conceptualizations, we lay complementary groundwork to facilitate coherence and critical understanding.

Racism

We define racism as the interconnected social, political, economic, and ideological systems that create, maintain, and exacerbate stratification in access to opportunities and resources based on a group's or individual's location in a socially constructed racial hierarchy (Bonilla-Silva 1997).[1] Social science literature identifies several key components of racism. Racialization is one fundamental component, illustrating the relational nature of racism. Through processes of racialization, societies establish differences between social groups, create boundaries between the groups, and assign differential value to these groups on the basis of race (Bonilla-Silva 1997; Omi and Winant 2015; Schwalbe et al. 2000). In turn, these processes create subordinate and dominant racial groups, and social actors and institutions leverage differential value to justify the stratification of life chances based on race (Bonilla-Silva 1997; Omi and Winant 2015; Schwalbe et al. 2000).

Across race-conscious societies, racism is context- and time-specific (Bonilla-Silva 1997). While systems of racial stratification have historical roots, they rely on contemporary processes to shape each racial group's position in the racial strata (Bonilla-Silva 1997). Though race is often the most salient social category in race-conscious societies, other social statuses and identities, such as gender, class, and nativity, also shape one's location in those racial strata and one's experiences of racism (Bonilla-Silva 1997; Collins 2015; Crenshaw 1991). Race is also a unit of identity and group membership (Bonilla-Silva 1997; Nagel 1994). Experiences of racism are not unidirectional: groups and individuals are continuously navigating racial classifications and racism, and they are working to assert, attenuate, resist, and/or transform racial categories and hierarchies.

Racism functions at multiple socioecological levels including across systems, institutions, and ideologies, and at the individual level (e.g., individual beliefs, behaviors, or practices) (Gee and Ford 2011; Jones 2000). Notably, racism can operate in the absence of individuals who perpetrate interpersonal racism (Bonilla-Silva 1997; Jones 2000). Accordingly, the elimination of racial inequities requires addressing structural racism: the interconnected systems, institutions, ideologies, and processes that create, preserve, and augment discriminatory ideologies and values and that in turn shape access to life chances and resources and that structure inequities across racial groups (Bailey, Feldman, and Bassett 2021; Bonilla-Silva 1997; Gee and Ford 2011; Jones 2000, 2003).

This special issue features scholarship focused on understanding how structural racism shapes conceptualization of the drivers of racial

1. Under the umbrella of "racism," we include related terms such as structural, institutional, and systemic racism. All these point beyond individual acts of discrimination or personal sentiments of prejudice and toward the systems and structures that perpetuate racial inequality (which include and rely on individual ideas and actions but amount to much more than the sum of those individual parts).

differences in health, the collection of public health data to inform the monitoring of racial health inequities, the politics of health outcomes, and the policies that affect health and well-being.

Health

In 1948, the World Health Organization defined health as "a state of complete physical, mental, and social well-being, and not merely the absence of disease or infirmity" (World Health Organization 2021). This oft-cited definition highlights the importance of a multidimensional understanding of health. Yet this definition still reflects Western medical models by characterizing "health" as the absence of a disease or illness.[2] Moreover, the World Health Organization's conceptualization of health focuses narrowly on the health of individuals, overlooking community and population health. In contrast, Indigenous definitions of health highlight the limits of medicalized conceptualizations. While definitions vary, notions of health articulated by indigenous communities often offer more holistic perspectives. Such definitions may link individual health with the well-being of family, kin networks, and community, and may incorporate the natural world and sociocultural factors into understandings of physical, mental, spiritual, and ecological well-being (Arquette et al. 2002).

In this special issue we view health as pertaining to individual, community, and population-level well-being, and we embrace conceptualizations of health as a process. Several of the empirical analyses featured in this special issue incorporate a life course perspective (Halfon and Hochstein 2002) that recognizes the embodiment of social inequities borne out of structural racism, the intergenerational transmission of embodied inequities, short- and long-term health outcomes, and how inequities may accumulate or intersect to shape health trajectories. Two articles in this special issue (Robinson and Pearlman 2021; Rodriguez et al. 2021) examine health outcomes that are highly sensitive to acute life events, such as birth outcomes. One study (Morey et al. 2021) chronicles cases of and deaths due to COVID-19, an emerging infectious illness that can have enduring physiological effects. Another study (LeBrón et al. 2021) explores how navigating racialized identities can shape mental and physical well-being in the short, intermediate, and longer term.

2. The COVID-19 pandemic may spur some theorists and practitioners to revisit this definition of health, particularly as a larger share of the population lives with the intermediate- and longer-term physical, mental, and social effects of COVID-19.

Politics

In addition to studying health as a process, the articles in this special issue demonstrate the value of approaching politics as a process. Though politics is often understood in terms of elections and voting, it is much more than an electoral or behavioral outcome. Politics is a process through which policies and other institutions shape a variety of life outcomes, including health. Political processes at the national, state, and local levels structure the economic and social outcomes that create (or impede) the conditions necessary for health. Politics directly influences core elements of the public health system (e.g., through appropriations, regulation, administration, subsidization), including the resources and human infrastructure necessary to support community-based prevention efforts; monitor the health of the population; address social determinants of health and health inequities; and develop and implement timely, robust, equity-centered interventions during public health crises. Politics also affects the health care system through myriad policies that impact health care workforces, health care organizations (e.g., hospitals, clinics), corporate actors (e.g., insurance providers, pharmaceutical companies), and more. Further still, political processes influence indirect factors that are critical to health and well-being, including the accessibility and generosity of social welfare benefits, the prevalence of conditions that threaten health (e.g., poverty, gun violence, air pollution, lead poisoning), and the cultivation of conditions that foster health (e.g., safe neighborhoods, clean air, broad access to social and material resources).

These political processes operate through a range of actors and governance institutions. Relevant actors include political elites (e.g., the president, state governors, state and local legislators), bureaucrats (at agencies such as the Centers for Disease Control and Prevention, the Food and Drug Administration, the Centers for Medicare and Medicaid Services, etc.), interest groups (e.g., hospital associations, health advocacy groups), and ordinary people. These and other actors operate within an array of institutions that shape and constrain their choices and behavior. Such institutions range from large and encompassing (political parties, federalism) to concentrated and focused (local health departments, "street level" public-serving bureaucracies, municipal governments, community-based organizations). Actors and institutions across these levels and venues drive political processes that shape health, and they do so in ways that are affected by structural racism, with marked implications for racial (in)equity. Examples of this abound. Federalism is a profoundly racialized institution (i.e., it reinforces processes of racial stratification), with consequences for health equity (Michener 2018). Political parties are also racialized institutions (Mason 2018; McDaniel and Ellison 2008; Philpot 2009, 2017; Valentino and Zhirkov 2018), with ramifications for the politics of health (Grumbach 2018; Henderson and Hillygus 2011; Morone 2016; Wilkes 2015; Rodriguez, Bound, and Geronimus 2014). Likewise, a wide variety of political actors engage with health politics in ways that have discernible implications for racial health (in)equity. This includes everyone from ordinary white Americans whose racial biases shape their attitudes toward Medicaid expansion and work requirements (Grogan and Park 2017; Haeder, Sylvester, and Callaghan 2021; Lanford and Quadagno 2016), to state governors who are more likely to be politically rewarded for expanding Medicaid when they govern states with larger populations of white Medicaid beneficiaries (Fording and Patton 2019), to policy makers who invest less in Medicaid enrollees with disabilities in states where levels of racial resentment are higher (Leitner, Hehman, and Snowden 2018), to Medicaid bureaucrats who treat Black Medicaid beneficiaries less fairly in hearings contesting their removal from the program (Franklin 2017).

In the face of such complexity, nuanced and systematic attentiveness to how health politics intersects with structural racism is crucial. One challenging imperative is to account for racism, health, and politics through integrated approaches that consider all three phenomena. The bulk of existing research emphasizes two of the three, at most. There are many studies that examine racism and health (Mateo and Williams 2021; Phelan and Link 2015; Williams and Collins 2001; Williams, Lawrence, and Davis 2019; Williams and Mohammed 2013). There is also an important corpus of research on racism and politics/policy (Bensonsmith 2005; Katznelson 2005; King and Smith 2005; Lieberman 1995, 1998, 2005; Matsubayashi and Rocha 2012; Michener 2019; Orloff 2002; Schram, Soss, and Fording 2010; Soss, Fording, and Schram 2011; Williams 2003). Finally, there is a strong and growing body of work on politics, policy, and health, much of which has been prominently featured in this journal (Carpenter 2012; Gollust and Haselswerdt 2019; Grogan and Patashnik 2003; Hacker and Skocpol 1997; Haselswerdt 2017; Haselswerdt and Michener 2019; Jacobs and Mettler 2011; Michener 2017; Oberlander 2001, 2003; Ojeda and Pachecho 2019; Pachecho and Fletcher 2015; Patashnik and Oberlander 2018).

Notwithstanding each of these distinct areas of analysis, it is comparatively uncommon for scholars to simultaneously emphasize race/racism, health, and politics/policy. Even scholars who do such work are often not aware of one another (as reflected in citation practices and as a result of disciplinary boundaries) and are not robustly engaged by scholars in other related areas; for example, scholars of health policy too easily overlook work related to racism and health policy (for notable examples of scholarship that does address work on racism and health policy, see Cruz Nichols, LeBrón, and Pedraza 2018a, 2018b; Grogan and Park 2017; Hooijer and King 2021; Kline 2019; Lanford and Quadagno 2021; LeBrón et al. 2018; LeBrón et al. 2019; Lopez 2019; Michener 2018, 2020; Pedraza, Cruz Nichols, and LeBrón 2017; Novak, Geronimus, and Martinez-Cardoso 2017; Young, Beltrán-Sánchez, and Wallace 2020). Putting this array of literatures and approaches into conversation and engagement with one another is an important step in producing knowledge useful for advancing health equity.

Interdisciplinary Approaches to Racism, Health, and Politics

The articles in this special issue draw on a range of disciplinary perspectives and methodological approaches to make substantive empirical and theoretical contributions at the nexus of racism, health, and politics. Chowkwanyun opens this special issue with a review of historical and contemporary analytic frameworks and tropes for understanding racial differences in health. This review highlights how explanatory frameworks held by scholars and practitioners shape discourse, research, and policy approaches to addressing population health inequities. By offering a critical analytical perspective on the concept of a "racial health disparity," Chowkwanyun helpfully unsettles the larger research ecosystem, pushing both scholars and practitioners to closely examine the first principles structuring their interpretive prisms.

Pivoting the emphasis of this special issue from concepts to data, Morey and colleagues illuminate how structural racism shapes the politics of being counted and categorized, demonstrating the consequences for the reporting of COVID-19 cases and deaths for Native Hawaiians and Pacific Islanders. Morey and colleagues discuss the role of racially color-blind policies in perpetuating failures of data collection and reporting, which in turn diminishes the chance to leverage data on racial health inequities to inform health equity efforts. Their analysis points not only to the importance of implementing policies designed to collect and report information about race and ethnicity but also to the imperative of monitoring and requiring compliance with such policies.

As this special issue turns to substantive analyses of how racialization processes affect health outcomes, Rodriguez, Bae, Geronimus, and Bound assess the linkages between federal- and state-level political parties in power and implications for Black-white inequities in birth outcomes. The authors argue that the partisan political agendas of US presidents and state legislatures have helped to maintain institutional racism that permeates the social determinants of health. Through quantitative empirical work, they articulate a historically and institutionally grounded analysis of racial differences in a critical health outcome. Ultimately, this research challenges readers to consider the idea that transforming US politics and its racialized nature is essential to promoting health equity.

In a complementary analysis, Robinson and Pearlman evaluate how social policy affects birth outcomes for Black and white mothers. They find that state spending on the earned income tax credit and state laws raising the minimum wage reduce the risk of low birthweight and preterm births for Black mothers (with a less consistent effect for white mothers). This work underscores the extent to which social and economic policies are public health interventions. Cash and in-kind transfer programs that benefit racially and economically marginalized populations can ameliorate racial inequities in the structural determinants of health. Even in a larger context of "bounded justice," where advances in health equity are limited by enduring institutional commitments to white supremacy and capitalism (Creary 2021), Robinson and Pearlman demonstrate the continued importance of a more generous and robust welfare state (Michener, SoRelle, and Thurston 2020).

This special issue closes with a methodological shift. Through a qualitative inquiry, LeBrón and colleagues examine immigration and immigrant policies as a form of structural racism that determines the opportunity to migrate to the US via authorized migration pathways, contributes to the long-standing and growing deportation regime against unauthorized immigrants, and restricts the rights of unauthorized and other immigrants. Analyzing data from interviews with immigrant and US-born Mexican-origin women, they trace how racialization occurs in a raced, classed, and gendered society and unfolds in ways that implicate political actors, systems, and policies. Instructive to both researchers and practitioners (e.g., advocates, organizers, policy makers), this study explores how Mexican-origin women respond to and navigate racialization processes, where they find agency and opportunity for action, and the short-, intermediate-, and long-term health implications thereof.

Looking Forward

Taken together, the papers in this special issue generate insights that other scholars can apply, critically assess, and build upon. This work is a springboard toward the continuing development of knowledge that advances the study of racism, health, and politics. With an eye toward such development, we conclude this introductory article with thoughts on directions for future thinking and research.

Populations, Topics, and Methodological Considerations

The study of racism, health, and politics in the United States is most advanced in understanding the health of Black Americans relative to white Americans (as the Robinson and Pearlman article in this special issue demonstrates). Yet, in addition to the enslavement and sustained oppression of people of African descent, the economic and political growth of the United States was also rooted in the genocide of Native peoples and the conquest of both Latin American and Polynesian territories. Thus, greater attention is needed to characterize and grasp the interconnections between racism, health, and politics for indigenous peoples, Latinas/os/xs/es, Asians, and Native Hawaiians and Pacific Islanders. This also includes necessary research on the health of racially minoritized groups who are currently classified as "white" by the standards of the Office of Management and Budget, such as Arab and Persian peoples.

In addition, research on health, racism, and politics requires recognizing the many complexities produced by long-standing practices and institutions of racial oppression. For example, scholars should attend to heterogeneity *within* racial categories, the importance of time and change (e.g., cohort studies, longitudinal research), the relevance of place-based processes of racialization, the significance of national or territorial origin or descent, and much more. Comparative analyses are especially critical: even as scholars expand the purview of research to more robustly include a wider range of racially minoritized groups, we might consider the function of anti-Blackness by juxtaposing health experiences and outcomes for Black people with those of other racially minoritized groups. Intersectional analyses are also essential. Intersectional perspectives account for the experiences of numerous social identities and positionalities (e.g., class, gender, sexuality)—identities that are multiplicative, not additive (Al-Faham, Davis, and Ernst 2019; Crenshaw 1991; Michener, Dilts, and Cohen 2012). Finally, the multiracial population in the United States is often omitted from studies of racism, health, and politics. Given the substantial growth of the multiracial population (Jones et al. 2021), studies of how racism shapes the politics and health of multiracial persons are long overdue (Davenport 2018).

On an institutional level of analysis, empirical studies are needed that capture dynamic and interconnected systems and processes that create, perpetuate, preserve, and/or reduce structural racism. This will require studying how structural racism operates and is upheld across multiple social and ecological levels and several dimensions of population health and via numerous mechanisms by which social inequities shape health simultaneously. Big data (e.g., health system, social media, and federally reported data) is often perceived as being well positioned to explore the role of multiple mechanisms and processes simultaneously. However, it is important to consider both the opportunities and the limitations of big data for capturing both the blunt and the stealthy ways in which structural racism operates as well as the unique and shared impacts for racially minoritized groups. Moreover, racism is contextually and temporally specific, taking on different shapes across time and place, and is influenced by historical and contemporary processes. Studies involving big data must grapple with how to incorporate these important components of racism into the analytic inquiry and data. More critical attention is needed to ways big data may further marginalize racially minoritized groups for whom data collection and reporting is problematic and/or cases where population sizes may be small. Additionally, we need more studies that investigate the health equity implications of political efforts to reduce structural racism, considering simultaneously the role of federal, state, and local processes in shaping health outcomes.

Reflecting the understanding that health is a process, the study of racism, health, and politics requires analysis of longitudinal and intergenerational data that illuminate how racism and politics shape health across the life course, and how health shapes racism and politics. Such studies have the potential to disentangle the role of time, temporality, and directionality in shaping when and how the health consequences of structural racism materialize in clinical indicators of health status, and how health shapes politics and policies.

This special issue brings into conversation scholarship representing researchers across disciplines such as political science, public health, ethnic studies, and economics, and it includes the voices of nonacademic scholars who are leaders of community-based efforts to address structural racism. The next generation of interdisciplinary scholarship on the study of racism, health, and politics must integrate multiple positionalities and disciplines to advance the science of interdisciplinary scholarship. This will require valuing, funding, and creating opportunities for cross-sector and cross-discipline exchange and collaboration, such as encouraging and supporting the publication of interdisciplinary scholarship; securing a commitment from journals to publish works that transcend disciplinary boundaries and provide adequate space to explain and unpack interdisciplinary concepts and analyses; ensuring that journal reviewers are equipped to assess the strengths and weaknesses of interdisciplinary scholarship as well as scholarship that studies the interconnections between racism, health, and politics; and rewarding scholars for publishing in interdisciplinary journals and/or outside of their fields.

Finally, what is the study of racism, health, and politics without attention to translating this knowledge into action? The effective translation of scholarship on racism, health, and politics will involve building the capacity of scholars to discuss, and even coproduce research findings with affected communities and policy designers; valuing and funding the investment in capacity-building and translational research efforts; and ensuring that scholarship is free and open access for community-based leaders and policy-making institutions.

Scientific research about health outcomes, health care systems, public health, health inequities, and other phenomena related to health and racism provides a necessary but insufficient foundation of knowledge. To facilitate change, politics and policy must also be incorporated into the purview of scholarly inquiry on health and racism. Knowledge about how politics and policy structure the relationships between racism and health is vital for understanding how to redress racism and thwart its devastating health consequences. Ida B. Wells-Barnett, a trailblazing journalist of the late 19th and early 20th centuries, famously said that "the way to right wrongs is to turn the light of truth upon them" (Wells 1892). This insight reverberates nearly 130 years later. Health inequities are a product of the persistent wrong of structural racism. We cannot change this wrong without seeing it clearly: its political causes and consequences, its policy mechanisms and repercussions, its material significance in the lives of racially marginalized communities. This special issue is a call for scholars across disciplines and traditions to further illuminate the wrong of structural racism, its effects on health and well-being, and the role of politics and policy in producing and/or mitigating those effects.

▪ ▪ ▪

Jamila Michener is an associate professor of government and public policy at Cornell University. She studies the politics of poverty, racism, and public policy in the United States. She is author of *Fragmented Democracy: Medicaid, Federalism and Unequal Politics* (2018). Prior to working at Cornell, she was a Robert Wood Johnson Health Policy Scholar at the University of Michigan.
jm2362@cornell.edu

Alana M. W. LeBrón is an assistant professor of health, society, and behavior and Chicano/Latino studies at the University of California, Irvine. Her scholarship focuses on mechanisms by which structural racism shapes the health of communities of color, with a focus on policies, systems, and environments. Much of her scholarship involves community-based participatory research, working in partnership with members of affected communities to strengthen understanding of the ways in which structural racism shapes health inequities and to develop and evaluate strategies that advocate for structural change, mitigate the health impacts of structural racism, and create new systems to promote health equity.
alebron@uci.edu

References

Akee, Randall, and Sarah Reber. 2021. "American Indians and Alaska Natives Are Dying of COVID-19 at Shocking Rates." February 18. www.brookings.edu/research/american-indians-and-alaska-natives-are-dying-of-covid-19-at-shocking-rates/.

Al-Faham, Hajer, Angelique M. Davis, and Rose Ernst. 2019. "Intersectionality: From Theory to Practice." *Annual Review of Law and Social Science* 15: 247–65.

Andrews, Kehinde. 2021. "Racism Is the Public Health Crisis." *Lancet* 397, no. 10282: P1342–43.

Arquette, Mary, Maxine Cole, Katsi Cook, Brenda LaFrance, Margaret Peters, James Ransom, Elvera Sargent, Vivian Smoke, and Arlene Stairs. 2002. "Holistic Risk-Based Environmental Decision Making: A Native Perspective." *Environmental Health Perspectives* 110, suppl. 2: 259–64.

Bailey, Zinzi D., Justin M. Feldman, and Mary T. Bassett. 2021. "How Structural Racism Works—Racist Policies as a Root Cause of US Racial Health Inequities." *New England Journal of Medicine* 384, no. 8: 768–73.

Bailey, Zinzi D., and J. Robin Moon. 2020. "Racism and the Political Economy of COVID-19: Will We Continue to Resurrect the Past?" *Journal of Health Politics, Policy and Law* 45, no. 6: 937–50.

Barber, Sharrelle. 2020. "Death by Racism." *Lancet Infectious Diseases* 20, no. 8: 903.

Barber, Sharrelle. 2021. "Silence Is No Longer an Option: Reflections on Racism and Resistance in the Midst of Coronavirus Disease 2019 Pandemic." *Epidemiology* 32, no 1: 133–34.

Bateman, David A., Ira Katznelson, and John S. Lapinski. 2018. *Southern Nation: Congress and White Supremacy after Reconstruction*. Princeton, NJ: Princeton University Press.

Bensonsmith, Dionne. 2005. "Jezebels, Matriarchs, and Welfare Queens: The Moynihan Report of 1965 and the Social Construction of African-American Women in Welfare Policy." In *Deserving and Entitled: Social Constructions of Public Policy*, edited by Anne L. Schneider and Helen M. Ingram, 243–60. Albany: State University of New York Press.

Blake, John. 2021. "There Was No Racial Reckoning." CNN, May 25. www.cnn.com/2021/04/18/us/george-floyd-racial-reckoning-blake/index.html.

Bonilla-Silva, Eduardo. 1997. "Rethinking Racism: Toward a Structural Interpretation." *American Sociological Review* 62, no. 3: 465–80.

Buchanan, Larry, Quoctrung Bui, and Jugal K. Patel. 2020. "Black Lives Matter May Be the Largest Movement in US History." *New York Times,* July 3.

Carpenter, Daniel. 2012. "Is Health Politics Different?" *Annual Review of Political Science* 15: 287–311.

Carter, Robert T., Michael Y. Lau, Veronica Johnson, and Katherine Kirkinis. 2017. "Racial Discrimination and Health Outcomes among Racial/Ethnic Minorities: A Meta-Analytic Review." *Journal of Multicultural Counseling and Development* 45, no. 4: 232–59.

Chowkwanyun, Merlin. 2022. "What Is a Racial Health Disparity? Five Analytic Traditions." *Journal of Health Politics, Policy and Law* 47, no. 2: 131–58.

Clinton, Joshua, Jon Cohen, John Lapinski, and Marc Trussler. 2021. "Partisan Pandemic: How Partisanship and Public Health Concerns Affect Individuals' Social Mobility during COVID-19." *Science Advances* 7, no. 2. doi.org/10.1126/sciadv.abd7204.

Collins, Patricia Hill. 2015. "Intersectionality's Definitional Dilemmas." *Annual Review of Sociology* 41: 1–20.

Creary, Melissa S. 2021. "Bounded Justice and the Limits of Health Equity." *Journal of Law, Medicine, and Ethics* 49, no. 2: 241–56.

Crenshaw, Kimberlé. 1991. "Mapping the Margins: Identity Politics, Intersectionality, and Violence against Women." *Stanford Law Review* 43, no. 6: 1241–99.

Cruz Nichols, Vanessa, Alana M. W. LeBrón, and Francisco I. Pedraza. 2018a. "Policing Us Sick: The Health of Latinos in an Era of Heightened Deportations and Racialized Policing." *PS: Political Science and Politics* 51, no. 2: 293–97.

Cruz Nichols, Vanessa, Alana M. W. LeBrón, and Francisco I. Pedraza. 2018b. "Spillover Effects: Immigrant Policing and Government Skepticism in Matters of Health for Latinos." *Public Administration Review* 78, no. 2: 432–43.

Davenport, Lauren D. 2018. *Politics beyond Black and White: Biracial Identity and Attitudes in America*. New York: Cambridge University Press.

Escobar, Gabriel J., Alyce S. Adams, Vincent X. Liu, Lauren Soltesz, Yi-Fen Irene Chen, Stephen M. Parodi, G. Thomas Ray, et al. 2021. "Racial Disparities in COVID-19 Testing and Outcomes: Retrospective Cohort Study in an Integrated Health System." *Annals of Internal Medicine* 174, no. 6: 786–93. doi.org/10.7326/M20-6979.

Fording, Richard C., and Dana J. Patton. 2019. "Medicaid Expansion and the Political Fate of the Governors Who Support It." *Policy Studies Journal* 47, no. 2: 274–99.

Franklin, Sekou. 2017. "The Politics of Race, Administrative Appeals, and Medicaid Disenrollment in Tennessee." *Social Sciences* 6, no. 1. doi.org/10.3390/socsci6010003.

Gadarian, Shana Kushner, Sara Wallace Goodman, and Thomas B. Pepinsky. 2021. "Partisanship, Health Behavior, and Policy Attitudes in the Early Stages of the COVID-19 Pandemic." *Plos One* 16, no. 4: doi.org/10.1371/journal.pone.0249596.

Gee, Gilbert C., and Chandra L. Ford. 2011. "Structural Racism and Health Inequities: Old Issues, New Directions." *DuBois Review: Social Science Research on Race* 8, no. 1: 115–32.

Gollust, Sarah E., and Jake Haselswerdt. 2019. "Health and Political Participation: Advancing the Field." *Journal of Health Politics, Policy and Law* 44, no. 3: 341–48.

Grogan, Colleen M., and Sunggeun Ethan Park. 2017. "The Racial Divide in State Medicaid Expansions." *Journal of Health Politics, Policy and Law* 42, no. 3: 539–72.

Grogan, Colleen, and Eric Patashnik. 2003. "Between Welfare Medicine and Mainstream Entitlement: Medicaid at the Political Crossroads." *Journal of Health Politics, Policy and Law* 28, no. 5: 821–58.

Grumbach, Jacob M. 2018. "From Backwaters to Major Policymakers: Policy Polarization in the States, 1970–2014." *Perspectives on Politics* 16, no. 2: 416–35.

Hacker, Jacob S., and Theda Skocpol. 1997. "The New Politics of US Health Policy." *Journal of Health Politics, Policy and Law* 22, no. 2: 315–38.

Haeder, Simon F., Steven M. Sylvester, and Timothy Callaghan. 2021. "Lingering Legacies: Public Attitudes about Medicaid Beneficiaries and Work Requirements." *Journal of Health Politics, Policy and Law* 46, no. 2: 305–55.

Hahn, Robert Alfred, Truman I. Benedict, and David R. Williams. 2018. "Civil Rights as Determinants of Public Health and Racial and Ethnic Health Equity: Health Care, Education, Employment, and Housing in the United States." *SSM—Population Health* 4: 17–24.

Halfon, Neal, and Miles Hochstein. 2002. "Life Course Health Development: An Integrated Framework for Developing Health, Policy, and Research." *Milbank Quarterly* 80, no. 3: 433–79.

Hardeman, Rachel R., Simone L. Hardeman-Jones, and Eduardo M. Medina. 2021. "Fighting for America's Paradise: The Struggle against Structural Racism." *Journal of Health Politics, Policy and Law* 46, no. 4: 563–75.

Haselswerdt, Jake. 2017. "Expanding Medicaid, Expanding the Electorate: The Affordable Care Act's Short-Term Impact on Political Participation." *Journal of Health Politics, Policy and Law* 42, no. 4: 667–95.

Haselswerdt, Jake, and Jamila Michener. 2019. "Disenrolled: Retrenchment and Voting in Health Policy." *Journal of Health Politics, Policy and Law* 44, no. 3: 423–54.

Henderson, Michael, and D. Sunshine Hillygus. 2011. "The Dynamics of Health Care Opinion, 2008–2010: Partisanship, Self-Interest, and Racial Resentment." *Journal of Health Politics, Policy and Law* 36, no. 6: 945–60.

Hooijer, Gerda, and Desmond King. 2021. "The Racialized Pandemic: Wave One of COVID-19 and the Reproduction of Global North Inequalities." *Perspectives on Politics*, August 11. doi.org/10.1017/S153759272100195X.

Hooper, Monica Webb, Anna María Nápoles, and Eliseo J. Pérez-Stable. 2020. "COVID-19 and Racial/Ethnic Disparities." *JAMA* 323, no. 24: 2466–67.

IOM (Institute of Medicine). 2003. *Unequal Treatment: Confronting Racial and Ethnic Disparities in Health Care*. Washington, DC: National Academies Press.

Jacobs, Lawrence R., and Suzanne Mettler. 2011. "Public Opinion, Health Policy, and American Politics: Editors' Introduction." *Journal of Health Politics, Policy and Law* 36, no. 6: 911–16.

Jones, Camara Phyllis. 2000. "Levels of Racism: A Theoretic Framework and a Gardener's Tale." *American Journal of Public Health* 90, no. 8: 1212–15.

Jones, Camara Phyllis. 2003. "Confronting Institutionalized Racism." *Phylon* 50, nos. 1–2: 7–22.

Jones, Nicholas, Rachel Marks, Roberto Ramirez, and Merarys Ríos-Vargas. 2021. "2020 Census Illuminates Racial and Ethnic Composition of the Country." US Census Bureau, August 12. www.census.gov/library/stories/2021/08/improved-race-ethnicity-measures-reveal-united-states-population-much-more-multiracial.html.

Katznelson, Ira. 2005. *When Affirmative Action Was White: An Untold History of Racial Inequality in Twentieth-Century America*. New York: W. W. Norton and Company.

King, Desmond S., and Rogers M. Smith. 2005. "Racial Orders in American Political Development." *American Political Science Review* 99, no. 1: 75–92.

Kline, Nolan. 2019. *Pathogenic Policing: Immigration Enforcement and Health in the US South*. New Brunswick, NJ: Rutgers University Press.

Kneipp, Shawn M., Todd A. Schwartz, Denise J. Drevdahl, Mary K. Canales, Sheila Santacroce, Hudson P. Santos Jr., and Ruth Anderson. 2018. "Trends in Health Disparities, Health Inequity, and Social Determinants of Health Research: A 17-Year Analysis of NINR, NCI, NHLBI, and NIMHD Funding." *Nursing Research* 67, no. 3: 231–41.

Lanford, Daniel, and Jill Quadagno. 2016. "Implementing Obamacare: The Politics of Medicaid Expansion under the Affordable Care Act of 2010." *Sociological Perspectives* 59, no. 3: 619–39.

Lanford, Daniel, and Jill Quadagno. 2021. "Identifying the Undeserving Poor: The Effect of Racial, Ethnic, and Anti-Immigrant Sentiment on State Medicaid Eligibility." *Sociological Quarterly*, February 25. doi.org/10.1080/00380253.2020.1797596.

LaVeist, Thomas A. 1992. "The Political Empowerment and Health Status of African-Americans: Mapping a New Territory." *American Journal of Sociology* 97, no. 4: 1080–95.

LeBrón, Alana M. W., Amy J. Schulz, Cindy Gamboa, Angela Reyes, Edna A. Viruell-Fuentes, and Barbara A. Israel. 2018a. "'They Are Clipping Our Wings': Health Implications of Restrictive Immigrant Policies for Mexican-Origin Women in a Northern Border Community." *Race and Social Problems* 10, no. 3: 174–92.

LeBrón, Alana M. W., Keta Cowan, William D. Lopez, Nicole L. Novak, Maria Ibarra-Frayre, and Jorge Delva. 2018b. "It Works, but for Whom? Examining Racial Bias in Carding Experiences and Acceptance of a County Identification Card." *Health Equity* 2, no. 1: 239–48.

LeBrón, Alana M. W., Keta Cowan, William D. Lopez, Nicole L. Novak, Maria Ibarra-Frayre, and Jorge Delva. 2019. "The Washtenaw ID Project: A Government-Issued ID Coalition Working toward Social, Economic, and Racial Justice and Health Equity." *Health Education and Behavior* 46, suppl. 1: 53S–61S.

LeBrón, Alana M. W., Ivy R. Torres, Enrique Valencia, Miriam López Dominguez, Deyaneira Guadalupe Garcia-Sanchez, Michael D. Logue, and Jun Wu. 2019. "The State of Public Health Lead Policies: Implications for Urban Health Inequities and Recommendations for Health Equity." *International Journal of Environmental Research and Public Health* 16, no. 6: 1–28.

LeBrón, Alana M. W., Amy J. Schulz, Cindy Gamboa, Angela Reyes, Edna Viruell-Fuentes, and Barbara A. Israel. 2022. "Mexican-Origin Women's Construction and Navigation of Racialized Identities: Implications for Health Amid Restrictive Immigrant Policies." *Journal of Health Politics, Policy and Law* 47, no. 2: 259–291.

Leitner, Jordan B., Eric Hehman, and Lonnie R. Snowden. 2018. "States Higher in Racial Bias Spend Less on Disabled Medicaid Enrollees." *Social Science and Medicine* 208: 150–57.

Lieberman, Robert C. 1995. "Race, Institutions, and the Administration of Social Policy." *Social Science History* 19, no. 4: 511–42.

Lieberman, Robert C. 1998. *Shifting the Color Line: Race and the American Welfare State*. Cambridge, MA: Harvard University Press.

Lieberman, Robert C. 2005. *Shaping Race Policy: The United States in Comparative Perspective*. Princeton, NJ: Princeton University Press.

Lopez, Leo, Louis H. Hart, and Mitchell H. Katz. 2021. "Racial and Ethnic Health Disparities Related to COVID-19." *JAMA* 325, no 8: 719–20.

Lopez, William D. 2019. *Separated: Family and Community in the Aftermath of an Immigration Raid*. Baltimore: Johns Hopkins University Press.

Lurie, Nicole. 2005. "Health Disparities—Less Talk, More Action." *New England Journal of Medicine* 353, no. 7: 727–29.

Mason, Lilliana. 2018. *Uncivil Agreement: How Politics Became Our Identity*. Chicago: University of Chicago Press.

Mateo, Camila M., and David R. Williams. 2021. "Racism: A Fundamental Driver of Racial Disparities in Health-Care Quality." *Nature Reviews Disease Primers*, March 11. doi.org/10.1038/s41572-021-00258-1.

Matsubayashi, Tetsuya, and Rene R. Rocha. 2012. "Racial Diversity and Public Policy in the States." *Political Research Quarterly* 65, no. 3: 600–14.

McDaniel, Eric L., and Christopher G. Ellison. 2008. "God's Party? Race, Religion, and Partisanship over Time." *Political Research Quarterly* 61, no. 2: 180–91.

Michener, Jamila. 2017. "People, Places, Power: Medicaid Concentration and Local Political Participation." *Journal of Health Politics, Policy and Law* 42, no. 5: 865–900.

Michener, Jamila. 2018. *Fragmented Democracy: Medicaid, Federalism, and Unequal Politics*. Cambridge: Cambridge University Press.

Michener, Jamila. 2019. "Policy Feedback in a Racialized Polity." *Policy Studies Journal* 47, no. 2: 423–50.

Michener, Jamila. 2020. "Race, Politics, and the Affordable Care Act." *Journal of Health Politics, Policy and Law* 45, no. 4: 547–66.

Michener, Jamila. 2021. "Politics, Pandemic, and Racial Justice through the Lens of Medicaid." *American Journal of Public Health* 111, no. 4: 643–46.

Michener, Jamila, Mallory SoRelle, and Chloe Thurston. 2020. "From the Margins to the Center: A Bottom-Up Approach to Welfare State Scholarship." *Perspectives on Politics*, November 10. doi.org/10.1017/S153759272000359X.

Michener, Jamila Celestine, Andrew Dilts, and Cathy J. Cohen. 2012. "African American Women: Intersectionality in Politics." In *The Oxford Handbook of African American Citizenship, 1865–Present*, edited by Henry Louis Gates Jr., Claude Steele, Lawrence D. Bobo, Michael Dawson, Gerald Jaynes, Lisa Crooms-Robinson, and Linda Darling-Hammod, 492–518. Oxford: Oxford University Press.

Morey, Brittany N., Richard Calvin Chang, Karla Blessing Thomas, 'Alisi Tulua, Corina Penaia, Vananh D. Tran, Nicholas Pierson, John C. Greer, Malani Bydalek, and Ninez Ponce. 2022. "No Equity without Data Equity: Data Reporting Gaps for Native Hawaiians and Pacific Islanders as Structural Racism." *Journal of Health Politics, Policy and Law* 47, no. 2: 159–200.

Morone, James A. 2016. "Partisanship, Dysfunction, and Racial Fears: The New Normal in Health Care Policy?" *Journal of Health Politics, Policy and Law* 41, no. 4: 827–46.

Nagel, Joane. 1994. "Constructing Ethnicity: Creating and Recreating Ethnic Identity and Culture." *Social Problems* 41, no. 1: 152–76.

Novak, Nicole L., Arline T. Geronimus, and Aresha M. Martinez-Cardoso. 2017. "Change in Birth Outcomes among Infants Born to Latina Mothers after a Major Immigration Raid." *International Journal of Epidemiology* 46, no. 3: 839–49.

Oberlander, Jonathan. 2001. "Medicare: Issues in Political Economy." *Journal of Health Politics, Policy and Law* 26, no. 1: 175–80.

Oberlander, Jonathan. 2003. *The Political Life of Medicare*. Chicago: University of Chicago Press.

Ojeda, Christopher, and Julianna Pacheco. 2019. "Health and Voting in Young Adulthood." *British Journal of Political Science* 49, no. 3: 1163–86.

Omi, Michael, and Howard Winant. 2014. *Racial Formation in the United States*. 3rd ed. New York: Routledge.

Ong, Paul, Chhandara Pech, Silvia Gonzalez, Sonja Diaz, Jonathan Ong, and Elena Ong. 2020. "Left Behind during a Global Pandemic: An Analysis of Los Angeles County Neighborhoods at Risk of Not Receiving Individual Stimulus Rebates under the CARES Act." UCLA Center for Neighborhood Knowledge and UCLA Latino Policy and Policy Initiative. latino.ucla.edu/wp-content/uploads/2020/04/LPPI-CNK-Brief-2-with-added-notes-res.pdf (accessed November 15, 2021).

Orloff, Ann Shola. 2002. "Explaining US Welfare Reform: Power, Gender, Race, and the US Policy Legacy." *Critical Social Policy* 22, no. 1: 96–118.

Pacheco, Julianna, and Jason Fletcher. 2015. "Incorporating Health into Studies of Political Behavior: Evidence for Turnout and Partisanship." *Political Research Quarterly* 68, no. 1: 104–16.

Patashnik, Eric M., and Jonathan Oberlander. 2018. "After Defeat: Conservative Postenactment Opposition to the ACA in Historical-Institutional Perspective." *Journal of Health Politics, Policy and Law* 43, no. 4: 651–82.

Pearlman, Jessica, and Dean E. Robinson. 2022. "State Politics, Racial Disparities, and Income Support: A Way to Address Infant Outcomes and the Persistent Black-White Gap?" *Journal of Health Politics, Policy and Law* 47, no. 2: 225–58.

Pedraza, Franciso I., Vanessa Cruz Nichols, and Alana M. W. LeBrón. 2017. "Cautious Citizenship: The Deterring Effect of Immigration Issue Salience on Health Care Use and Bureaucratic Interactions among Latino US Citizens." *Journal of Health Politics, Policy and Law* 42, no. 5: 925–60.

Phelan, Jo C., and Bruce G. Link. 2015. "Is Racism a Fundamental Cause of Inequalities in Health?" *Annual Review of Sociology* 41: 311–30.

Philpot, Tasha S. 2009. *Race, Republicans, and the Return of the Party of Lincoln*. Ann Arbor: University of Michigan Press.

Philpot, Tasha S. 2017. *Conservative but Not Republican: The Paradox of Party Identification and Ideology among African Americans*. New York: Cambridge University Press.

Pirtle, Whitney N. 2020. "Racial Capitalism: A Fundamental Cause of Novel Coronavirus (COVID-19) Pandemic Inequities in the United States." *Health Education and Behavior* 47, no. 4: 504–8.

Putnam, Lara, Erica Chenoweth, and Jeremy Pressman. 2020. "The Floyd Protests Are the Broadest in US History—And Are Spreading to White, Small-Town America." *Washington Post*, June 6.

Rodriguez, Javier M., Byengseon Bae, Arline T. Geronimus, and John Bound. 2022. "The Political Realignment of Health: How Partisan Power Shaped Infant Health in the United States, 1915–2017." *Journal of Health Politics, Policy and Law* 47, no. 2: 201–24.

Rodriguez, Javier M., John Bound, and Arline T. Geronimus. 2014. "US Infant Mortality and the President's Party." *International Journal of Epidemiology* 43, no. 3: 818–26.

Rothstein, Richard. 2017. *The Color of Law: A Forgotten History of How Our Government Segregated America*. New York: Liveright Publishing.

Schram, Sanford F., Joe Brian Soss, and Richard Carl Fording, eds. 2010. *Race and the Politics of Welfare Reform*. Ann Arbor: University of Michigan Press.

Schwalbe, Michael, Daphne Holden, Douglas Schrock, Sandra Godwin, Shealy Thompson, and Michele Wolkomir. 2000. "Generic Processes in the Reproduction of Inequality: An Interactionist Analysis." *Social Forces* 79, no. 2, 419–52.

Smedley, Brian D., Adrienne Y. Stith, and Alan R. Nelson, eds. 2003. *Unequal Treatment: Confronting Racial and Ethnic Disparities in Healthcare*. Washington, DC: National Academies Press.

Snowden, Lonnie, and Genevieve Graaf. 2019. "The 'Undeserving Poor,' Racial Bias, and Medicaid Coverage of African Americans." *Journal of Black Psychology* 45, no. 3: 130–42.

Soss, Joe, Richard C. Fording, and Sanford F. Schram. 2011. *Disciplining the Poor: Neoliberal Paternalism and the Persistent Power of Race*. Chicago: University of Chicago Press.

Valentino, Nicholas A., and Kirill Zhirkov. 2018. "Blue Is Black and Red Is White? Affective Polarization and the Racialized Schemas of US Party Coalitions." Paper presented at the Midwest Political Science Association Conference, Palmer House Hilton, Chicago, April 5–8.

Vestal, Christine. 2020. "Racism Is a Public Health Crisis, Say Cities and Counties." *Stateline* (blog), June 15. www.pewtrusts.org/en/research-and-analysis/blogs/stateline/2020/06/15/racism-is-a-public-health-crisis-say-cities-and-counties.

Wailoo, Keith. 2014. *Dying in the City of the Blues: Sickle Cell Anemia and the Politics of Race and Health*. Chapel Hill: University of North Carolina Press.

Wallerstein, Nina. 1992. "Powerlessness, Empowerment, and Health: Implications for Health Promotion Programs." *American Journal of Health Promotion* 6, no. 3: 197–205.

Washington, Harriet A. 2006. *Medical Apartheid: The Dark History of Medical Experimentation on Black Americans from Colonial Times to the Present*. New York: Doubleday Books.

Wells, Ida Barnett. 1892. "Miss Ida B. Wells, a Lecture." *Washington Bee*, October 22.

Williams, David R., and Chiquita Collins. 2001. "Racial Residential Segregation: A Fundamental Cause of Racial Disparities in Health." *Public Health Reports* 116, no. 5: 404–16.

Williams, David R., Jourdyn A. Lawrence, and Brigette A. Davis. 2019. "Racism and Health: Evidence and Needed Research." *Annual Review of Public Health* 40: 105–25.

Williams, David R., and Selina A. Mohammed. 2013. "Racism and Health I: Pathways and Scientific Evidence." *American Behavioral Scientist* 57, no. 8: 1152–73.

Williams, Linda Faye. 2003. *The Constraint of Race: Legacies of White Skin Privilege in America*. University Park, PA: Penn State University Press.

Wilkes, Rima. 2015. "We Trust in Government, Just Not in Yours: Race, Partisanship, and Political Trust, 1958–2012." *Social Science Research* 49: 356–71.

World Health Organization. 2021. "Constitution." www.who.int/about/governance/constitution (accessed August 16, 2021).

Yearby, Ruqaiijah, Crystal N. Lewis, Keon L. Gilbert, and Kira Banks. 2020. "Memo: Racism Is a Public Health Crisis. Here's How to Respond." Data for Progress (blog), September 3. www.dataforprogress.org/memos/racism-is-a-public-health-crisis.

Young, Maria-Elena de Trinidad, Hiram Beltrán-Sánchez, and Steven P. Wallace. 2020. "States with Fewer Criminalizing Immigrant Policies Have Smaller Health Care Inequities between Citizens and Noncitizens." *BMC Public Health* 20, no. 1: 1–10.

Zelner, Jon, Rob Trangucci, Ramya Naraharisetti, Alex Cao, Ryan Malosh, Kelly Broen, Nina Masters, and Paul Delamater. 2021. "Racial Disparities in Coronavirus Disease 2019 (COVID-19) Mortality Are Driven by Unequal Infection Risks." *Clinical Infectious Diseases* 72, no. 5: e88–95. doi.org/10.1093/cid/ciaa1723.

Zimmerman, Frederick J., and Nathaniel W. Anderson. 2019. "Trends in Health Equity in the United States by Race/Ethnicity, Sex, and Income, 1993–2017." *JAMA Network Open* 2, no. 6: e196386. doi.org/10.1001/jamanetworkopen.2019.6386.

What Is a "Racial Health Disparity"? Five Analytic Traditions

Merlin Chowkwanyun
Columbia University

Abstract What exactly is a "racial health disparity"? This article explores five lenses that have been used to answer that question. It contends that racial health disparities have been presented—by researchers both within academia and outside of it—as problems of five varieties: biology, behavior, place, stress, and policy. It also argues that a sixth tradition exploring class—and its connection to race, racism, and health—has been underdeveloped. The author examines each of these conceptions of racial disparities in turn. Baked into each interpretive prism is a set of assumptions about the mechanisms that produce disparities—a story, in other words, about where racial health disparities come from. Discursive boundaries set the parameters for policy debate, determining what is and is not included in proposed solutions. How one sees racial health disparities, then, influences the strategies a society advocates—or ignores—for their elimination. The author ends by briefly discussing problems in the larger research ecosystem that dictate how racial health disparities are studied.

Keywords racial health disparities, racial equity, racism and health

More than 35 years ago, the US Department of Health and Human Services (HHS) published an eight-volume report on "Black and Minority Health" (HHS 1985). Dubbed the "Heckler Report" (after Secretary of Health and Human Services Margaret Heckler), it was a comprehensive survey of racial disparities, offering data on overall mortality, health care access, the racial composition of health personnel, maternal and child health, violence, and chronic disease. The report was an analogue to *An American Dilemma*, the Swedish economist Gunnar Myrdal's exhaustive 1944 study on racism in the United States (Myrdal 1944). The chair of the task force

Journal of Health Politics, Policy and Law, Vol. 47, No. 2, April 2022
DOI 10.1215/03616878-9517163

that assembled the Heckler Report declared that it would be "a generating force for an accelerated national assault on . . . persistent health disparities."

Whatever its shortcomings, the Heckler Report signaled federal recognition of racial health disparities as a core public health priority. It led to the creation of the Office of Minority Health in HHS, and it sparked research that culminated in the National Institute on Minority Health and Health Disparities. A 2019 special supplement published by that agency showcased new ways of measuring racial health disparities, evaluating interventions to ameliorate them, and establishing causation and understanding their impacts over a person's life course (Jones et al. 2019), all refined over the decades. As David R. Williams, Jourdyn Lawrence, and Brigette Davis (2019) put it in an *Annual Review of Public Health* field survey published that same year, this "body of research illustrates the myriad ways in which the larger social environment can get under the skin to drive health and inequities in health." Nearly four decades after Heckler, it is worth taking stock of where the field has come and where it might go.

Rather than cover every crevice of the field, I instead focus on a simple question: "What exactly is a racial health disparity?" I take a cue from writers who have probed the nature of "poverty" (Gans 1972; Katz 2015; O'Connor 2001). Like a racial health disparity, poverty on its surface is simple: a blunt metric of deprivation. Yet this simplicity masks contestation about its causes, ways to eliminate it, and above all, its fundamental essence. Is poverty fundamentally a problem of an individual's cumulative life choices? Is it a by-product of the geographic location where one is born or lives? Or is it rooted in the larger economic system in which one must survive? In short, what kind of a problem, as the late social critic Michael B. Katz asked, is poverty?

I contend that racial health disparities have been interpreted and explained—by researchers both within academia and outside of it—as problems of five kinds: biology, behavior, place, stress, and policy. The politics of some of these five analytic traditions have not always been straightforward and, indeed, were sometimes embraced by partisans of divergent ideological persuasions. They were also shaped by the vicissitudes of history. For most of the 20th century, explanations for racial health disparities were deeply reactionary and outright racist, but after the civil rights revolution of the 1960s, alternatives to reigning accounts had more space to flourish. These new explanatory narratives, however, did not fully situate racial health disparities in the larger political-economic order. Class, I conclude, is a sixth way of problematizing racial health disparities that remains underdeveloped in American analyses.

I proceed with three caveats. First, although the most common population comparison made in the examples that follow is between Black and white people, that fact reflects emphases in the discourse, particularly academic literature. But as some other examples show, the five analytic traditions are still marshaled when the health of other non-Black racialized populations has been under discussion. Second, I do not focus on nomenclature and debate over using the term "disparities" as opposed to others such as "inequalities" or "inequities." I use "disparities" simply because it remains commonplace, even as writers have increasingly identified flaws with this phraseology, particularly with regard to what they see as lack of a "fairness judgment" (Braveman 2014; Hammonds and Reverby 2019; Lynch and Perera 2017). Last, I present these traditions as distinct. My purpose in doing so is not to depict a false mutual exclusivity. Rather, I am conveying the core kernel of each tradition, illustrated with real-world examples in which one overriding constitutive factor shapes explanations of racial health disparities more than others. From this list of five analytic traditions, readers will find other examples where the traditions operate in tandem and in more varied ways.

This is not a typological exercise for its own sake. As with poverty, a freestanding and seemingly objective quantitative indicator of a racial health disparity obscures the multiple optics one can bring to explaining the world—and the racism within it—that produced the figure (Espeland and Stevens 2008). Baked into each interpretive prism is a set of assumptions about the mechanisms that produce disparities—a story, in other words, about where racial health disparities come from. As Julie Lynch and Isabel Perera note (2017), such discursive boundaries set the parameters for policy debate, determining what is and is not included in proposed solutions. How one sees racial health disparities, then, influences the strategies a society advocates—or ignores—for their elimination.

Methods

I identified the five traditions by reviewing three types of publications: public health and social science research on racial disparities; primary source writings published in various time periods examining the relationship between race and health; and historical scholarship on race and American medicine, science, and public health. I constructed a corpus through a combination of means: using various keyword permutations and combinations (e.g., "race," "disparities," "racial," "ethnic," "health," "inequalities," "inequities") and entering them into the PubMed database;

following references in highly cited articles; and drawing on my own knowledge of the historical scholarship. For analysis, I mostly read inductively, identifying notions of what caused racial health disparities. If they recurred in the corpus itself and were invoked by contemporaries for at least two decades, I declared the notion an analytic tradition. I identified the underdeveloped sixth tradition—class—by considering adjacent literatures on social class and health, general racial stratification, and theoretical social science explicitly examining the race-class nexus.

Racial Health Disparities as a Problem of Biology

For most of American history, differential health outcomes were interpreted as by-products of a supposed natural hierarchy of biologically discrete races. Even when successfully challenged at various junctures, these explanations have endured.

In the antebellum period, physicians characterized enslaved people as prone to various behaviors, such as eating dirt; immune to certain diseases; or having weaker organs (Heller 1995; Hogarth 2017; Willoughby 2017). By the late nineteenth century, these discourses persisted in a more elaborated body of scientific knowledge, in which various indices of biological difference—measures of brains, lungs, skulls, and others—were cited to explain gradients in health. This practice was bolstered by new statistical techniques for capturing characteristics of population groups, plus growing knowledge of genetics, each of which allowed racist ideology to assume an objective and scientific gloss (Gould [1981] 1996; Zuberi 2003). The idea of multiple discrete human origins and evolutionary paths that mapped onto biologically rooted racial hierarchy circulated in mainstream scientific thinking as well (Stocking 1968). Known as polygenism, this idea provided further fuel for explaining racial health disparities as immutable natural facts.

The new racial science served unique American political ends, especially with the consolidation of Jim Crow in 1896. It not only justified state-sanctioned discrimination in a variety of spheres, from public accommodations to labor markets to housing options, but also turned explanations for poor Black health away from resource scarcity and toward supposedly innate traits of the formerly enslaved themselves. Assessing a widely circulated publication about "race traits" that argued respiratory capacity was lower in Black people than in white people, W. E. B. Du Bois captured this orientation away from society toward individual biology, stating that the tract's author "finally concludes that the cause of the failure of so many peoples in the struggle of life is the lack of those race characteristics for which the Aryan is pre-eminent" (Du Bois 1897, Wolff 2006).

A parallel discourse emerged around immigrants. It gained traction as record immigration to the United States in the 1890s raised anxieties about labor competition and societal change brought on by the incursion of newcomers from eastern and southern Europe and East Asia. Often, expressions of public health threat simply pointed to outsiderness. But increasingly, this discourse became explicitly hereditarian, especially when espoused by eugenicists, with some groups deemed more fit and others more "feeble-minded" and weak (Kevles [1985] 1995). Political discourse fixated on the "fecundity" of immigrants and how they might retard the national birth rate. Such concerns about the biological constitution of newcomers arose amid nativism that culminated in the Immigration Act of 1924, which imposed stringent country-specific quotas and banned Asian immigration altogether (Ngai 1999).

But the biological race concept and attendant notions of inferiority came under severe challenge after World War I. From anthropology came studies by Franz Boas that partially undermined prevailing biological classifications (Baker 1998; Yudell 2014). The so-called "first" UNESCO Statement on Race declared in 1950 that "race is less a biological fact than a social myth and as a myth it has in recent years taken a heavy toll in human lives and suffering" (UNESCO 1969), and its chief author was Ashley Montagu, who had authored *Man's Most Dangerous Myth* ([1942] 1974) a decade earlier. A seminal paper by the population geneticist Richard Lewontin (1972) found that 85% of genetic variation occurred within so-called "races," not across them, undercutting the case for biological races and, by extension, the health disparities that could be explained away by them.

Yet racial biology never died a clean death. The 1950 UNESCO statement was attacked by many in the scientific establishment, and a second revision qualified its core claims (Brattain 2007). Many geneticists, like Theodore Dobzhansky, accepted most of the criticism leveled at the biological race concept but still had trouble relinquishing the notion entirely (Yudell 2014). The notion was similarly alive in public health research, most notoriously in the Tuskegee syphilis experiments, which were predicated on the belief that the disease developed differently in Black people (Reverby 2009). At century's end, racial biology anchored openly racist books such as Charles Murray and Richard Herrnstein's *The Bell Curve* (1994), which argued for the existence of congenital racial differences in intelligence.

In the late 1990s and early 2000s, novel genome sequencing techniques and completion of the Human Genome Project injected new life into claims that races were biological. Geneticist Neil Risch proclaimed that new data from a study he led showed that commonsensical racial categories indeed had a genetic basis (Risch, Burchard, Ziv, and Tang 2002; Tang et al. 2005). Some scientists offered terms like "admixture" to move beyond traditional and discrete racial categories, but they ultimately still anchored observed group differences in biology (Fullwiley 2008; Rajagopalan and Fujimura 2012).

In medicine, scholars demonstrated that biological race concepts—old and new—crept up in routine literature and were regularly used to explain racial health disparities in breast cancer, respiratory disease, and other conditions. They expressed concern that in clinical practice, race might be used as a blunt—and erroneous—proxy for assessing a patient and prescribing differential treatment (Braun et al. 2007). Race correction, the practice by which a different "normal" reference range is used for diagnosing Black patients, was premised on biological race. It attracted increasing criticism by scholars (Braun et al. 2020) but remained widely used and taught with no consensus as yet on whether the practice should cease. Meanwhile, the billion-dollar market for ancestry detection kits reinforced notions of biological race in the popular imagination (Bolnick et al. 2007).

One notable aspect of racial biology's twenty-first-century resurrection was that it proceeded not under the guise of racial animus, as it had a century prior, but instead racial egalitarianism. The marketing of BiDil—a heart drug whose manufacturer claimed it would have particular effectiveness in Black patients—was defended on the grounds that it would close the gap in cardiac racial health disparities (Kahn 2014). And Esteban Burchard, an expert on racial health disparities in asthma, has argued that some of these disparities are rooted in pharmacological differences between racial groups' response to medications (Aldhouse 2016). For him, eradicating racial health disparities meant searching for genetic roots. If it once looked like racial health disparities as a problem of a biology had become a thing of the past, the present moment has left that conclusion in sharp doubt.

Racial Health Disparities as a Problem of Behavior

An equally durable explanation for racial health disparities was behavior. Here again, Jim Crow and nativism were turning points. By the late nineteenth century, newspapers and public health inspection reports regularly asserted that certain lifestyles were endemic to particular racial groups. These dispatches came with an exoticizing gaze that focused on supposedly elevated levels of substance abuse, unhygienic living habits, and inability to follow health dictates. One inspector in San Francisco's Chinatown, for example, wrote in 1885 that "the mode of life among the Chinese here are [sic] not much above those of rats on the waterfront" (Shah 2001). African Americans in Baltimore were frequently characterized as "incorrigible consumptives" by physicians and nurses overseeing tuberculosis campaigns, with similarly lurid descriptions of their homes and purportedly race-specific habits (Roberts 2009). As with biology, behavioral narratives made individuals the central unit of analysis, not social subordination and its role in poor health outcomes.

Behavioral analyses were not always the provenance of racists. But they could still be shot through with middle-class moralism. Du Bois's 1899 *Philadelphia Negro*, for example, did not escape fixations, prevalent in the settlement house movement, on nonnormative family structure and what Du Bois called the "laxity in morals" allegedly arising from Black migrants' adjustment to city life in the north (Du Bois 1899; Hartman 2020; Reed 1997). Some civil rights organizations, such as the Urban League (Reed 2008), similarly focused on the perceived inability of constituents to embrace proper social mores, part of what Kevin Gaines (1996) has called an "uplift ideology" common among middle-class African American civic leaders of the time. Many immigrants rallied behind a strategy of outward decorum and respectability as well. In the 1930s, Nayan Shah (2001) notes, Chinese American advocates for public housing argued that it would facilitate stable nuclear families and shield them from the lifestyles of vice-ridden Chinese bachelors who lived unhealthily and elsewhere.

In the 1960s, behavior assumed center stage in larger social policy debate. Daniel Patrick Moynihan's *The Negro Family: The Case for National Action* (1965) centered on Black households without male heads, which led, in the author's view, to a "tangle of pathology" that mired African Americans in poverty and unemployment. In the 1980s, some analysts and public officials claimed that public assistance incentivized dependency (Katz 2013). Both the Moynihan report and subsequent welfare reform rhetoric led to criticism from those who pointed out what they perceived to be racist and sexist overtones and assumptions.

These criticisms also informed contemporary public health approaches. Increasingly few practitioners of health promotion completely divorced "health behaviors" from larger social networks, living conditions, and life circumstances in which people lived. Yet there was no doubt, as a look through a highly used health promotion textbook indicated, that there existed an uneasy tension between frameworks that focused on how an individual cycled through various cognitive states and frameworks that took a more social-ecological view of why some people were more likely—and had the means—to behave in health-reinforcing ways (Glanz, Rimer, and Viswanath 2015). This was especially the case in the field of immigrant health, which continued to center heavily around "acculturation" and whether it contributed to helpful or harmful health behaviors, such as the adoption of certain diets or substance use (Lara et al. 2005).

The behavioral tradition held up in the public sphere as well. In 2010, Annice Kim and colleagues studied racial health disparities discourse in the broader public sphere (Kim et al. 2010). Analyzing a decade of newspaper coverage, they found that African Americans were most frequently centered and that the leading explanation offered for disparities was behavioral (versus "societal"). Furthermore, behavioral solutions accounted for "nearly half" of those foregrounded by the articles examined.

Nevertheless, awareness of stigma—and its frequently racialized underpinnings—grew enormously among both scholars and practitioners in the first two decades of the 21st century. Behavioral explanations lacked the flagrantly pathologizing quality that they had had a century prior. But narrow conceptions of racial health disparities as a problem of behavior still persisted, even as the larger field had long pursued more holistic explanations. It is to those we now turn.

Racial Health Disparities as a Problem of Space

If biology and behavior were influential but incomplete—and sometimes erroneous—explanations for racial health disparities, what other arenas did the field explore? One was space: the exploration of differential location by race and its health effects. In the United States, Du Bois's *Philadelphia Negro* (1899) was an exemplar of this analysis. On health and other metrics of wellness, it documented white–Black mortality and morbidity differentials not just in the aggregate but ward by ward. Du Bois advanced beyond European studies of spatial difference and health by also incorporating the role of ascriptive difference (Coleman 1982; Jones-Eversley and Dean 2018). Indeed, Du Bois might well have been the first entry in the spatial tradition of racial health disparities work.

Du Bois wrote in 1899. Unfortunately, for much of the ensuing century, space proved to be a rather Janus-faced optic. In fact, for the first two thirds of the 20th century, it was more often deployed for destructive ends. The racial segregation of immigrants and African Americans led to what one scholar has labeled "territorial stigmatization" (Wacquant 2007). At the turn of the century, public officials frequently depicted immigrant and Black neighborhoods as cauldrons of contagious disease and a threat to cities at large, providing rationales for racial segregation and even destruction of unhealthy areas (Molina 2006; Roberts 2009; Shah 2001).

These local-level actions scaled up in the middle of the century with the advent of the federal urban renewal program. In 1948, the American Public Health Association's Committee on Hygiene and Health developed rubrics to determine whether neighborhoods ought to be razed if they were deemed enough of a public health hazard. In Russ Lopez's (2009) words, these scales "supplied a scientific and seemingly impartial justification for declaring a neighborhood blighted." They also gave cities across the country "a procedure for targeting neighborhoods for destruction," one backed by the public health profession, that forcibly relocated selected inhabitants away from more affluent residents to whom their living quarters had posed an alleged risk.

The civil rights era, however, catalyzed new spatial thinking. Whereas previous incarnations examined threats to those *outside* segregated areas, subsequent analysis focused on the harms done to those *within* such neighborhoods. The sociologist Pierre De Vise, at the time head of the Chicago Regional Hospital Study, systematically documented links between residential segregation and health services scarcity. He argued that Chicago's reputation as a medical powerhouse was belied by the way it treated Black patients. In an analysis of what he called the city's "apartheid health system," De Vise noted that four public hospitals were all concentrated in one section of town, necessitating onerous travel for those who depended on them. Of Cook County Hospital's patients during the previous year, "half had no health insurance of any kind, and nine-tenths were black. The average waiting time was two hours." By contrast, in other city hospitals, only "one-fifth had no insurance, and half were black."

At an even more granular level, De Vise examined neighborhoods with a sharp decline in white population and an increase in Black population. He found a precipitous drop in physician presence—by between 70% and 90%—as a neighborhood became more Black (De Vise 1971). Entire pockets of Chicago, then, were becoming medical deserts. De Vise's bleak portrait of Chicago mirrored that of cities like Los Angeles. There, the 1964 Watts uprising had spotlighted severe resource shortfalls in south central Los Angeles, leading a commission to call for the construction of a full-service hospital there (Viseltear 1967). If midcentury medicine was a story of boom and technological accomplishment, these reports were a reminder that it had advanced along geographically and racially segregated lines.

This research was limited in one fundamental way: "health" meant health care. Subsequent academic research on residential segregation evolved in capacious ways. One branch, pioneered by figures such as Thomas LaViest (1989), Chiquita Collins (with David Williams, 1999), and David Williams (with Chiquita Collins, 2001), explored the association between residential segregation and health in a broader sense, captured by aggregate indices such as low birth weights and infant and all-cause mortality. Later, studies appeared about specific illnesses, including cancer, diabetes, and cardiovascular disease. In general, the more segregated an area was, the worse its health outcomes were.

It was harder, however, to move from strong ecological association to a more specific articulation of the pathway between racial composition of a neighborhood and the health of individuals within it. But other work on neighborhood effects offered some answers, exploring the health consequences of geographically concentrated advertising for harmful products, limited walkability, nonavailability of certain foods, and lack of social service supports (Roux 2001). These were not solely problems in racially segregated neighborhoods, but often they were most pronounced in such areas, especially when tied to simultaneous economic hardship.

Other scholars turned to place-specific analysis. One of the most ambitious attempts came from those who examined Detroit, most of them based at the University of Michigan. Their studies walked a taut line: coming up with generalizable propositions on the one hand, while anchoring phenomena in local characteristics unique to a place on the other. The work stood out for the way it frequently situated its findings in Detroit's history of deindustrialization, white exodus, declining tax bases, and pervasive racial segregation (Schulz et al. 2002). The Detroit work did not depend exclusively on large national secondary datasets; it also drew on surveys conducted by the venerable Detroit Area Study, and occasionally, more granular data obtained by partnering with community-based groups. Besides neighborhood effects, the Detroit studies also explored the impact of decentralized city government, the city's labor market, and pollution.

Most spatially oriented research did not identify a single overriding mechanism tying segregation and health. Rather, it offered multiple, sometimes more hypothetical, pathways threading economics, race, and geography. One exception was environmental justice research. Here, the argument was forthright and direct: a major cause of racial health disparities, especially in respiratory and cardiovascular illnesses, came from toxicological hazards—bus depots, garbage dumps, highways, factories—disproportionately located in low-income minority neighborhoods.

Activists had long noted these patterns in cities large and small (Hurley 1995). But documentation of these patterns had not quite coalesced into a more systematic formal body of knowledge. That changed in the 1980s, with a series of lawsuits arguing that unequally distributed environmental burdens amounted to civil rights violations. A growing body of spatial research, much of it synthesized in Robert Bullard's *Dumping in Dixie* (1990), showed strong associations between adverse environmental health outcomes and racial composition of an area. Much of the work came from unusually fruitful academic partnerships with community groups, with the former supplying technical assistance and the latter providing on-the-ground knowledge about where to even look for potential risks. One early collaboration—still in existence—that drew attention from both environmental health advocates and researchers was between Columbia University's Center for Environmental Health in northern Manhattan and the West Harlem Environmental Action Network (Minkler, Vásquez, and Shepard 2006; Sze 2007). It focused on air quality issues connected to diesel fuel and the high concentration of bus depots in the area. On the other side of the country, the Southern California Environmental Justice Collaborative connected local organizations and foundations with three academic institutions—the University of California at Santa Cruz, Occidental College, and Brown. The academic partners worked to analyze publicly available data, which community organizations subsequently used to lobby successfully for better regional emissions standards. These collaborations did not just exist in large cities. In Ottawa County, Oklahoma, Native American advocates worked with researchers from Emory University, the University of Oklahoma, and the University of New Mexico to document children's elevated lead levels stemming from hazardous construction projects. Dubbed Tribal Efforts Against Lead, the collaboration gave lay residents input into the study design and provided them with evidence of serious health risks in areas where Native Americans resided (Minkler et al. 2006).

The elegance of the environmental justice narrative did conceal some ambiguities behind the patterns its champions had documented. Did the phenomena result from planners' racial antipathy toward residents themselves? Did the problems arise from policy makers' perception that political reaction from the most powerless would be muted when it came to locational choices? What role did economics—and the tendency of polluters to cluster hazards on cheap land—play alongside residential segregation?

The answers to these questions could be complex. But to residents affected and their advocates, they were often scholastic and beside the point. In many regions, from New York City to Anniston, Alabama, racial minorities bore the greatest brunt of pollution, whatever the cause, and the goal was to establish this outcome's existence, then mitigate its effects. Efforts in the courtroom and at the grassroots level paid off in 1994, when President Bill Clinton signed an executive order mandating that federal agencies "identify and address" actions of theirs that might result in the unequal environmental health burdens. It affirmed a core claim of not just environmental justice but the spatial tradition: that geographic arrangements produced racial health disparities.

Racial Health Disparities as a Problem of Stress

If spatial analyses were highly ecological, another school of thinking focused on societal-to-physiological pathways. Racial health disparities here were conceptualized as a problem of accumulated stress. The most agenda-setting work was conducted by Sherman James in the early 1980s. James created a scale to measure "John Henryism," named after a retired African American sharecropper in North Carolina whom James had met and who had worked himself to near exhaustion under trying lifelong circumstances (1993). John Henryism measured one's commitment to "hard work" and perseverance, especially in the face of adversity.

The general pattern James uncovered in his work was as follows: high levels of John Henryism in African American men were associated with alarming cardiovascular consequences, namely blood pressure levels and hypertension (James et al. 1984; James et al. 1987; James, Hartnett, and Kalsbeek 1983). Moreover, the effect was far more pronounced in those of lower socioeconomic status and did not typically hold for white men. Heavy exertion in the face of substantial social impediments created a psychosocial reaction. Or, as James put it in a reflection on his work, "the combination of high stress (now significantly correlated with low socioeconomic status) and prolonged, high-effort coping with such stress is probably responsible for this strong elevation in risk" (1994). James's work explored larger settings in which people were embedded, particularly the workplace. The general association, he found, was strongest when one focused on lower-prestige occupations (James et al. 1984). It suggested that foreclosed opportunity and racial discrimination on the job were critical forces at play.

Arline Geronimus, a colleague of James's, elaborated on his questions. In studies on maternal and child health, she found that African American mothers who gave birth at younger ages had children with better health outcomes (measured by birth weight and mortality) than their older African American counterparts (Geronimus 1992, 1996). Geronimus hypothesized a temporal element in African American health, suggesting earlier onset of aging and physiological deterioration in Black versus white mothers. As did James, Geronimus suspected this acceleration was rooted in "psychosocial" stress and dubbed the phenomenon "weathering," posing it as a possible explanation for why *younger* Black mothers and their children in Geronimus's studies experienced fewer problems during childbirth.

Geronimus's work on racism and weathering grew more methodologically sophisticated. Her later studies used allostatic load (AL) scores: an aggregate measure of "chronic dysregulation (i.e., over-activity or inactivity) of physiological systems" as a result of repeated stressful events (McEwen and Gianaros 2010). Work on AL had uncovered strong associations between high scores and a host of undesirable health outcomes. Now, Geronimus applied its insights to racial health disparities. Using the AL measure with a number of large panel datasets, she suggested that typical physiological deterioration might occur sooner in African Americans than in whites because of the larger amount of external stressors African Americans confronted throughout their lives. The results could be dramatic—dispiritingly so. Models showed higher predicted Black AL scores (versus predicted white AL scores) in all age groups, especially in the adult years (Geronimus et al. 2006). On average, these models suggested that the onset of aging processes would take place an alarming 10 years earlier for African Americans than for whites. If racial health disparities were a problem of stress, they did not just come as ephemeral shocks at single points of time; rather, their effects accumulated, wearing and tearing one down over the years.

The exact external stressors at work were sometimes more implied than explicit. Everyday acts of racial discrimination and John Henryism were obvious ones. Elsewhere, Geronimus argued that her findings were not just the results of distressing person-to-person encounters. They stemmed from larger societal arrangements, including increasingly punitive social welfare policy and larger cultural stereotypes about African American single mothers, resulting in a public pathologization of this population—a practice that Geronimus outspokenly criticized (Geronimus 2000). Like James, Geronimus also explored the attenuating and amplifying effects of other axes of inequality. One was socioeconomic status (SES), where she found protective effects against Black mortality but less for morbidity (Geronimus 1992). Another found "nonpoor Blacks have a greater probability of high [allostatic load] scores than do poor Whites," disturbing evidence for how powerful stress effects could be (Geronimus et al. 2006).

A third set of important contributions to the stress tradition came from the Coronary Artery Risk Development in Young Adults (CARDIA) study, a longitudinal dataset started in 1985. One of its most creative users was Nancy Krieger, who deployed CARDIA to explore racial disparities in blood pressure. But whereas James had used John Henryism as a key input, Krieger used self-reported discrimination. Her findings could be complicated. Although moderate amounts of discrimination led to higher levels of blood pressure, one striking discovery was that those who reported no discrimination exhibited the highest levels of blood pressure. For Krieger, this was potential evidence of a stress effect resulting from a situation where "unfair treatment is perceived by members of stigmatized groups as 'deserved' and nondiscriminatory." Self-blame and denial, rooted in larger social stigmatization, thus manifested in stress and physiological consequences (Krieger and Sidney 1996). Another CARDIA study examined perinatal risk and odds of low birth weights, as Geronimus had done. It found that racial discrimination was associated with more than half of preterm deliveries and low birth weights among Black women compared to only 5% of preterm deliveries and 0% of low birth weights among white women (Mustillo et al. 2004). Here again, "racial discrimination as a psychosocial stressor" was the key factor at play.

Whatever input was used—John Henryism, AL scores, self-reported racial discrimination—the stress tradition found generally consistent results when it came to disparity, notwithstanding the occasional deviation from expected patterns. As generative as the findings themselves were, though, they also represented something else: a repudiation of the biological tradition. Stress research explored biological consequences—there was a surface similarity—but it started from the opposite premise of the field's forebears, who saw racial health disparities stemming from race as biological fact. The stress tradition, by contrast, held that racial health disparities were socially produced, the result of bodily coping with racism in its many manifestations. Geronimus and Krieger's attention to gender—and James's attention to the workplace setting—was strikingly prescient, too. Not only did it situate individual physiological deterioration in larger social contexts, its multifactorial nature also presaged what is now commonly dubbed "intersectional" analysis, long before the term became scholarly vogue.

Racial Health Disparities as a Problem of Policy

State-sponsored action—that is, public policy—was a final lens for analyzing racial health disparities. Policy has lurked under all the previous sections above. Racial biology and eugenics gave way to immigration restriction and residential segregation, as did widely held beliefs about the unhealthy group-specific behaviors of immigrants and African Americans. Contemporary spatial organization resulted from past land-use policies, leading later generations to debate what might reverse, at least partially, their deleterious effects on health. The stress research, though more implicitly than explicitly, pointed to lax enforcement of antidiscrimination laws and racially inflected welfare policy as sources of stressors.

These other traditions, however, did not explicitly *center* policy. For those who did, the most obvious site was health care access. Like most public and private accommodations in the United States, health care in the 20th century was racially segregated. This was entrenched by the 1946 Hill-Burton Act, which appropriated $75 million for building hospitals, 93% of which went to former Confederate states (McBride 1991; Thomas 2011). While it brought Southern health care services into closer line with the rest of the nation, it did so under Jim Crow logic. Many facilities were either all white or all Black, and those that were not remained racially segregated by ward.

It was not just hospitals, either. Most Black medical students attended Howard University College of Medicine and Meharry Medical College and were rarely admitted to other institutions, blocking wider African American entry into the profession. And after graduation, African American physicians were typically shut out of the state and local medical societies that were critical to gaining hospital privileges, leaving them professionally marginalized. Despite these constraints, Black hospitals and medical professionals—especially nurses and midwives—made significant strides in public health education and programming (Smith 1995).

In the 1950s, growing initiatives across the country documented local medical exclusion and linked it to racial health disparities. They coalesced into a broad civil rights coalition focused on desegregation of health care. In the words of David McBride, "an assertive black medical leadership believed that only confrontational civil-rights politics would in the end win black America's fight against the social diseases of poverty and racism, as well as the bodily diseases caused by infections and physical and mental debility" (1991). For them, racial health disparities were a problem of policy, stemming from legally sanctioned segregation.

Desegregation policy took many forms. The first was legal victories. In *Simkins v. Cone* (1963), the US Supreme Court declared segregated hospitals unconstitutional. But big-ticket legal precedents were only as good as enforcement. It would take two pieces of federal legislation, passed within a year of each other, to really affect circumstances on the ground. One was perhaps the most consequential law passed in the United States after World War II: the Civil Rights Act of 1964, which banned discrimination in both private and public spheres. The second was the passage of legislation creating Medicare and Medicaid. These new funds promised millions of dollars to health care facilities, which could now bill the government for services rendered to elderly and low-income patients. But Medicare and Medicaid also provided a big stick to break Jim Crow medicine. The federal government, civil rights activists reasoned, could threaten to withhold funds from facilities unless they complied with both high court rulings and new laws. Soon, the Department of Health, Education, and Welfare under President Lyndon Johnson implemented a sweeping inspections program to ensure facilities were in compliance. They did so under activist pressure from organizations like the National Medical Association, which represented the nation's Black physicians and patients, and the Medical Committee for Human Rights, an ad hoc organization created to provide medical assistance to civil rights workers in the South. The fight for desegregation of facilities had spillover consequences, too. It ended medical society segregation along with overtly exclusionary medical school admissions policies (Burrows and Berney 2019).

The consequences of desegregation, subsequent research has demonstrated, could be enormous. One analysis, by economist Douglas Almond and colleagues (2006), showed that after the onset of desegregation, mortality rates declined for Black infants much more sharply than for white infants, while racial health disparities narrowed. These trends were most pronounced in the rural South, where Jim Crow consolidation often blockaded access to health care services. There, the disparity was halved, with a decline of 11.4 deaths per 1,000 births, an astonishing fall that saved 4,000 lives in the decade after the new civil rights regime began. Explaining their findings, the authors pointed out that rapid treatments for pneumonia and gastroenteritis, two leading causes of infant death, were now no longer denied. Medicaid may also have contributed by financing African American access to health care institutions. A similar analysis performed by Nancy Krieger and colleagues (2013) found a striking convergence in Black infant mortality rates between "Jim Crow polities" and the rest of the country, one that began in the early 1970s and did not reverse until the end of the 20th century, though it never returned to pre-1970s levels. For the authors, this was evidence that "abolition of Jim Crow laws has contributed to shaping US infant death rates," in this case for the better.

Access to medical care nonetheless had a two-sided quality. A literature on physician bias, for example, uncovered discriminatory beliefs among white physicians toward nonwhite patients. One disturbing set of studies found that physicians sometimes assumed Black patients could naturally bear higher amounts of pain (Hoffman et al. 2016). Conceiving of racial health disparities as a problem of biology continued in formal medical knowledge (Braun et al. 2007). At worst, this could mean differential assessments of otherwise similar patients, skewed by beliefs about the role of a patient's race.

The demographic makeup of the medical profession was also slow to change, with historically underrepresented minorities still making up low percentages of entering classes. Even the entrance of women—a major positive reversal—masked underlying racial disparities: in 2015 only 7% of graduating women physicians were Black, and only 5% were Hispanic (Chowkwanyun and Howell 2019). The larger consequences of these phenomena for racial health disparities were less clear. But it underscored that removal of formal obstacles to medical institutions did not eliminate unequal dynamics within them. Likewise, beyond personnel, access could sometimes be theoretical, as shown by persistently higher rates of noninsurance in Black and Latino populations compared to whites, even as they were dramatically reduced by the Affordable Care Act, with the Black–white and Hispanic–white disparities falling by 4% and 8%, respectively (Buchmueller and Levy 2020).

For all the success of civil rights policy in the medical sphere, it never eliminated racial health disparities for a number of outcomes. To take just one example, from the field of maternal child health, the striking disparity in Black–white maternal deaths persisted and gained striking attention in the 2020 campaign cycle. It raised a question: was health care policy alone the chief domain to concentrate on when it came to racial health disparities? This concern was anchored in a larger classic question in public health about how much medical care actually contributed to population health improvement and group-to-group health disparities. More conservative estimates put the figure at around only 10%; more generous ones put it at around 50% (Cutler, Rosen, and Vijan 2006; Williams and Collins 1995). Either way, health care itself was clearly not the full story. Neither was the realm of the nonbiomedical, including factors identified by those in the spatial and stress traditions, such as racial prejudice, residential segregation, and environmental health hazards.

The importance of the social has led many concerned with racial health disparities to move outside not just the health care domain but health entirely for policy solutions. This was the vision of Health in All Policies (HiAP), an increasingly popular framework that many policy makers embraced to combat health disparities (Hall and Jacobson 2018). Its premise was simple: to better consider the health ramifications of domains not strictly labeled "health," such as housing, transportation, criminal justice, agriculture, and others. For instance, rather than solely designing bus routes to reduce transport time, a planner ought to also consider how rerouting buses might reduce or increase pollution in certain areas, and furthermore, whether any burdens might be disproportionately absorbed by racial minorities. Those designing new housing developments, to take another example, might incorporate health-abetting features—green spaces, walkways, convenient outlets for better foods—often absent in under-resourced and segregated areas. Some HiAP proponents have advocated using formal tools, such as health impact assessments (HIAs), to translate the notion into real-world practice. Like environmental impact assessments, HIAs provide a method to project the health ramifications of potential policies, including differential racial impacts (Collins and Koplan 2009). When used by those who work outside the formal health sector, they have the effect of rendering visible the health consequences of nonhealth policies.

Racial Health Disparities as a Problem of Class

One final dimension shaping disparities was class. Racial health disparities scholarship sat alongside a parallel literature on "social class" gradients in health, some of it produced by the same researchers (Krieger, Williams, and Moss 1997; Link and Phelan 1995). It drew from a sociological literature that sought to operationalize one's economic position—how to, for example, characterize white-collar professionals as a class. And it probed many important questions: whether it was best to measure SES as a single whole or break it out into income, education, and occupational components; the limits of the SES notion itself; how to incorporate occupational prestige; and the role of income inequality in health.

Yet when this research was brought to bear on racial health disparities, class's role could sometimes be simplified. Analysts took one of three courses. The first was to treat class—measured by a quantitative measure of SES—as a variable to be "controlled" against others. More often than not, class had some effect but did not eradicate racial health disparities entirely. A second was to stratify the study population by class and race.

The result generally showed that racial disparities endured, regardless of what level of class was examined. A third approach was to use interaction terms. This frequently demonstrated that lower economic class exacerbated racial health disparities.

These analyses were conducted in the language of econometrics and epidemiology. Here, class became a numeric metric conveying economic standing, while race was an ascriptive characteristic. One concluded which variable was more or less at work when it came to a particular racial health disparity. More sophisticated analyses factored in multiple levels of geography and other axes of difference such as gender. But for all their quantitative sophistication, much like "risk factor" analysis (Aronowitz 1998) that dominated much of the health sciences, they flattened dynamic social processes into tables and coefficients, mechanically isolating variables and their respective roles. And most of the time, they treated race and class as separate variables to be squared off against each other, rather than interstitial ones that shaped each other. This was true, too, of analysts who sought to explain racial health disparities by claiming they were primarily epiphenomenal effects of economic gulfs. What resulted were reams of data pointing to one or another variable's relative importance but not to the dynamic social contexts and institutional configurations that made it so.

A richer conception of class could be found in a longstanding literature on the race/class dynamic, rooted in the contributions of African American social scientists (almost all based in historically Black colleges) during the 1930s and 1940s (Cox 1948; Holloway 2002). Like the social class work, this school saw class not as a simple numeric indicator but as an individual's position relative to a labor system: that is, what sector a person worked in and whether the person received a wage or not, owned an enterprise (and if so, a small firm or a large one), operated inside or outside of formal labor markets, and so forth. This school also saw class as embedded in a dynamic system of institutions and social relations reconfigured from epoch to epoch.

Race, in this conception, came into being as an ideological construct used to rationalize New World societies' increasing dependence on enslaved people of African descent. With slavery's abolition came a reconfiguration of class relations; race continued to play a profound role, sorting the population into occupational hierarchies, and in the case of the Jim Crow United States, denying access to a host of accommodations, public programs, and occupational and residential options (Fields 1990; Morgan 1975; Wacquant 2002). For these scholars, the chief analytic goal was understanding how race operated differently as surrounding social relations changed.

The transformation of the race and class dynamic after Jim Crow and in the 21st century holds many potential implications for racial health disparities. Our approaches to understanding them must take into account many new developments. Consider just a handful. One is a massive upward distribution of income and wealth, datable to the mid-1970s and documented most vividly by economist Thomas Piketty (2013). A second is the breakdown in union membership, an overall retrenchment of a more robust welfare state, and the rise of austerity politics and budgetary stringency (Phillips-Fein 2017). This has particular ramifications for racial inequality, given the critical role of the public sector in facilitating stable and remunerative jobs for racial minorities after the civil rights movement (Katz, Stern, and Fader 2005; Pitts 2011).

Yet another is change in the very makeup of the labor force and the population at large. A Black–white binary has become increasingly untenable, with immigrants and their children making up larger demographic percentages in the United States and displacing white majorities altogether in certain states and municipalities. With demographic change has also come much more frequent use of nonwhite, non-Black racial identifiers and subidentifiers (e.g., foreign-born, third-generation, mixed-race, and so forth). This will challenge, in turn, the very definition and measurement of racial health disparities, which typically still rely on a default white reference group and assumptions about its average standing. A fourth and related development is the emergence of not interracial but intraracial economic inequality. Increasing stratification within racial categories undercuts how much race alone can signify about life chances, health and otherwise. (Katz and Stern 2006). While the rise of a Black professional class has received significant scholarly and policy attention (Boyd 2008; Lacy 2007; Pattillo 1999; Wilson 1987) for decades, a downwardly mobile—and drastically so—section of the white population has only recently generated significant interest (Case and Deaton 2015; Montez and Zajacova 2013). Its health ramifications are currently the subject of considerable debate, sparked by high-profile studies documenting declining white life expectancy.

A fifth, and final, development is capital movement (Cowie 1999; Self 2003; Souther 2017; Sugrue 1996), which has proceeded in waves since World War II and completely remade certain localities, hollowing out industrial cores and shrinking occupational opportunities in their wake, much of it felt most strongly by Black residents in cities like Camden, Detroit, Oakland, and Cleveland. The latest phase is technology that has upended entire sectors and consigned workers, many of them immigrants, to transient, low-wage service labor.

Each of these transformations comes with many potential adverse effects, many of which will be disproportionately felt by immigrants and African Americans, and will, by extension, adversely affect their health, especially those in the most marginal and subordinated of class positions. Figuring out the exact ways this will happen will be the task of future racial health disparities researchers.

Conclusion

For most of the 20th century, two ways of explaining racial health disparities—biology and behavior—were predominant, often at the expense of pathologized minorities. Three alternatives—what I have called the spatial, stress, and policy traditions—arose but came with their own internal tensions and limitations. Class analysis was present but often worked from a truncated and static notion of the term. Yet if the Great Recession of 2008 and the COVID-19 pandemic of 2020–21 have shown us anything, it is that the world of work and labor and the larger system of social relations is changing rapidly and undergoing continued upheaval. In addition to the robust spatial, stress, and policy traditions, class should better be incorporated in future racial health disparities discourse as a major analytic tradition. How might this occur?

Analyzing epoch-defining changes has mostly been left to qualitative social scientists and historians. These scholars' strength has been to identify precise agents, policies, and on-the-ground details that name the pieces of the system and how they operate. Their weakness, however, is limited familiarity and facility with the large-scale quantitative data of public health researchers. There is a real opportunity for cross-disciplinary collaboration and methodological complementarity here. Yet institutional structures and traditional funding agencies continue to privilege certain types of data and methods. They favor quantitative assessments of racial health disparities and interventions to reduce them, thereby devaluing studies that do not approach the problem from evaluative perspectives or statistical methods.

Thus, beyond adding or subtracting analytic traditions, it may be time to aim for more holism and methodological diversity in how we study health and why some attain well-being much more than others, especially along racial lines. For if our "long decade" of crises from 2008 to 2020 carries a single message, it is that now is no longer the time for scholarly business as usual.

■ ■ ■

Merlin Chowkwanyun is the Donald H. Gemson Assistant Professor in the Mailman School of Public Health at Columbia University. His work centers on the history of community health, environmental health regulation, racial inequality, and social movement/activism around health. His book *All Health Politics Is Local: Community Battles for Medical Care and Environmental Health* is forthcoming, and his current book project focuses on political unrest at medical schools and neighborhood health activism during the 1960s and 1970s.
mc2028@cumc.columbia.edu

Acknowledgments

My analytic debt to poverty scholars Herbert J. Gans, Alice O'Connor, Adolph L. Reed Jr., and Michael B. Katz should be obvious here. I also want to thank Alana LeBrón, Jamila Michener, Jon Oberlander, and the anonymous reviewers for their helpful comments. For an extremely probing and careful reading of an earlier draft, I thank Mo Torres.

References

Aldhouse, Peter. 2016. "Meet the Scientists Fighting for More Studies on Genes and Racial Differences in Health." *BuzzFeed News*, May 11. www.buzzfeednews.com/article/peteraldhous/science-so-white.

Almond, Douglas, Kenneth Chay, and Michael Greenstone. 2006. "Civil Rights, the War on Poverty, and Black-White Convergence in Infant Mortality in the Rural South and Mississippi." MIT Department of Economics, Working Paper No. 07–04, December 31. hdl.handle.net/1721.1/63330.

Aronowitz, Robert A. 1998. "The Social Construction of Coronary Heart Disease Risk Factors." In *Making Sense of Illness: Science, Society, and Disease*, 111–44. Cambridge: Cambridge University Press.

Baker, Lee. 1998. *From Savage to Negro: Anthropology and the Construction of Race, 1896–1954*. Berkeley: University of California Press.

Bolnick, Deborah A., Duana Fullwiley, Troy Duster, Richard S. Cooper, Joan H. Fujimura, Jonathan Kahn, Jay S. Kaufman, et al. 2007. "The Science and Business of Genetic Ancestry Testing." *Science* 318, no. 5849: 399–400.

Boyd, Michelle. 2008. *Jim Crow Nostalgia: Reconstructing Race in Bronzeville*. Minneapolis: University of Minnesota Press.

Brattain, Michelle. 2007. "Race, Racism, and Antiracism: UNESCO and the Politics of Presenting Science to the Postwar Public." *American Historical Review* 112, no. 5: 1386–413.

Braun, Lundy, Anne Fausto-Sterling, Duana Fullwiley, Evelynn M. Hammonds, Alondra Nelson, William Quivers, Susan M. Reverby, and Alexandra E. Shields. 2007. "Racial Categories in Medical Practice: How Useful Are They?" *PLOS Medicine*, September 25. doi.org/10.1371/journal.pmed.0040271.

Braun, Lundy, Anna Wentz, Reuben Baker, Ellen Richardson, and Jennifer Tsai. 2020. "Racialized Algorithms for Kidney Function: Erasing Social Experience." *Social Science and Medicine*, November 23. doi.org/10.1016/j.socscimed.2020.113548.

Braveman, Paula. 2014. "What Are Health Disparities and Health Equity? We Need to Be Clear." *American Journal of Public Health* 129, suppl. 2: 5–8.

Buchmueller, Thomas, and Helen Levy. 2020. "The ACA's Impact on Racial and Ethnic Disparities in Health Insurance Coverage and Access to Care." *Health Affairs* 39, no. 3: 395–402.

Bullard, Robert. 1990. *Dumping in Dixie: Race, Class, and Environmental Quality*. New York: Routledge.

Burrows, Vanessa, and Barbara Berney. 2019. "Creating Equal Health Opportunity: How the Medical Civil Rights Movement and the Johnson Administration Desegregated US Hospitals." *Journal of American History* 105, no. 4: 885–911.

Case, Anne, and Angus Deaton. 2015. "Rising Mortality and Morbidity among White Non-Hispanic Americans in the 21st Century." *PNAS* 112, no. 49: 15078–83.

Chowkwanyun, Merlin, and Benjamin Howell. 2019. "Health, Social Reform, and Medical Schools—The Training of American Physicians and the Dissenting Tradition." *New England Journal of Medicine* 381, no. 19: 15078–83.

Coleman, William. 1982. *Death Is a Social Disease: Public Health and Political Economy in Early Industrial France*. Madison: University of Wisconsin Press.

Collins, Chiquita, and David Williams. 1999. "Segregation and Mortality: The Deadly Effects of Racism?" *Sociological Forum* 14, no. 3: 495–523.

Collins, Janet, and Jeffrey Koplan. 2009. "Health Impact Assessment: A Step Toward Health in All Policies." *JAMA* 302, no. 3: 315–17.

Cowie, Jefferson. 1999. *Capital Moves: RCA's Seventy-Year Quest for Cheap Labor*. Ithaca, NY: Cornell University Press.

Cox, Oliver. 1948. *Caste, Class, and Race: A Study in Social Dynamics*. New York: Doubleday.

Cutler, David, Allison Rosen, and Sandeep Vijan. 2006. "Value of Medical Innovation in the United States: 1960–2000." *New England Journal of Medicine* 355, no. 9: 920–27.

De Vise, Pierre. 1971. "Cook County Hospital: Bulwark of Chicago's Apartheid Health System and Prototype of the Nation's Public Hospitals." *Antipode* 3, no. 1: 9–20.

Du Bois, W. E. B. 1897. "Review of Race Traits and the American Negro." *Annals of the American Academy of Political and Social Science*, July 1. doi.org/10.1177/000271629700900108.

Du Bois, W. E. B. 1899. *The Philadelphia Negro: A Social Study*. Philadelphia: University of Pennsylvania Press.

Espeland, Wendy, and Mitchell Stevens. 2008. "A Sociology of Quantification." *European Journal of Sociology* 49, no. 3: 401–36.

Fields, Barbara J. 1990. "Slavery, Race, and Ideology in the United States of America." *New Left Review* 1, no. 181: 95–118.

Fullwiley, Duana. 2008. "The Biologistical Construction of Race: 'Admixture' Technology and the New Genetic Medicine." *Social Studies of Science* 38, no. 5: 695–735.

Gaines, Kevin. 1996. *Uplifting the Race: Black Leadership, Politics, and Culture in the Twentieth Century.* Chapel Hill: University of North Carolina Press.

Gans, Herbert J. 1972. "The Positive Functions of Poverty." *American Journal of Sociology* 78, no 2: 275–89.

Geronimus, Arline. 1992. "The Weathering Hypothesis and the Health of African-American Women and Infants: Evidence and Speculations." *Ethnicity and Disease* 2, no. 3: 207–21.

Geronimus, Arline, 1996. "Black/White Differences in the Relationship of Maternal Age to Birthweight: A Population-Based Test of the Weathering Hypothesis." *Social Science and Medicine* 42, no. 4: 589–97.

Geronimus, Arline. 2000. "To Mitigate, Resist, or Undo: Addressing Structural Influences on the Health of Urban Populations." *American Journal of Public Health* 90, no. 6: 867–72.

Geronimus, Arline, Margaret Hicken, Danya Keene, and John Bound. 2006. "'Weathering' and Age Patterns of Allostatic Load Scores among Blacks and Whites in the United States." *American Journal of Public Health* 96, no. 5: 826–33.

Glanz, Karen, Barbara Rimer, and K. Viswanath, eds. 2015. *Health Behavior: Theory, Research, and Practice*. 5th ed. New York: Jossey-Bass.

Gould, Stephen J. (1981) 1996. *The Mismeasure of Man*. New York: W. W. Norton and Company.

Hall, Richard, and Peter Jacobson. 2018. "Examining Whether the Health-in-All-Policies Approach Promotes Health Equity." *Health Affairs* 37, no. 3: 364–70.

Hammonds, Evelynn, and Susan Reverby. 2019. "Toward a Historically Informed Analysis of Racial Health Disparities since 1619." *American Journal of Public Health* 109, no. 10: 1348–49.

Hartman, Sadiya. 2020. *Wayward Lives, Beautiful Experiments: Intimate Histories of Social Upheaval*. New York: W. W. Norton and Company.

Heller, John S. 1995. *Outcasts from Evolution: Scientific Attitudes of Racial Inferiority, 1859–1900.* Carbondale, IL: Southern Illinois University Press.

HHS (US Department of Health and Human Services). 1985. *Report of the Secretary's Task Force on Black and Minority Health.* Washington, DC: US Government Printing Office.

Hoffman, Kelly, Sophie Trawalter, Jordan Axt, and M. Norman Oliver. 2016. "Racial Bias in Pain Assessment and Treatment Recommendations, and False Beliefs about Biological Differences between Blacks and Whites." *PNAS* 113, no. 16: 4296–301.

Hogarth, Rana A. 2017. *Medicalizing Blackness: Making Racial Difference in the Atlantic World, 1780–1840.* Chapel Hill: University of North Carolina Press.

Holloway, Jonathan. 2002. *Confronting the Veil: Abram Harris, Jr., E. Franklin Frazier, and Ralph Bunche, 1919–1941*. Chapel Hill: University of North Carolina Press.

Hurley, Andrew. 1995. *Class, Race, and Industrial Pollution in Gary, Indiana, 1945–1980.* Chapel Hill: University of North Carolina Press.

James, Sherman. 1993. "The Narrative of John Henry Martin." *Southern Cultures* 1, no.1: 83–106.

James, Sherman. 1994. "John Henryism and the Health of African-Americans." *Culture, Medicine, and Psychiatry* 18: 163–82.

James, Sherman, Sue Hartnett, and William Kalsbeek. 1983. "John Henryism and Blood Pressure Differences among Black Men." *Journal of Behavioral Medicine* 6, no. 3: 259–78.

James, Sherman, Andrea LaCroix, David Kleinbaum, and David Strogatz. 1984. "John Henryism and Blood Pressure Differences among Black Men. II. The Role of Occupational Stressors." *Journal of Behavioral Medicine* 7, no. 3: 259–75.

James, Sherman, David Strogatz, Steven Wing, and Diane Ramsey. 1987. "Socioeconomic Status, John Henryism, and Hypertension in Blacks and Whites." *American Journal of Epidemiology* 126, no. 4: 664–73.

Jones, Nancy L., Nancy Breen, Rina Das, Tilda Farhat, and Richard Palmer, eds. 2019. "New Perspectives to Advance Minority Health and Health Disparities Research." Special issue, *American Journal of Public Health* 109, suppl.1.

Jones-Eversley, Sharon, and Lorraine Dean. 2018. "After 121 Years, It's Time to Recognize W. E. B. Du Bois as a Founding Father of Social Epidemiology." *Journal of Negro Education* 87, no. 3: 230–45.

Kahn, Jonathan. 2014. *Race in a Bottle: The Story of BiDil and Racialized Medicine in a Post-Genomic Age.* New York: Columbia University Press.

Katz, Michael B. 2013. *The Undeserving Poor: America's Enduring Confrontation with Poverty.* 2nd ed. New York: Oxford University Press.

Katz, Michael B. 2015. "What Kind of a Problem Is Poverty?" In *Territories of Poverty: Rethinking North and South,* edited by Ananya Roy and Emma Shaw Crane, 39–78. Athens: University of Georgia Press.

Katz, Michael B., and Mark J. Stern. 2006. *One Nation Divisible: What America Was and What It Is Becoming.* New York: Russell Sage Foundation.

Katz, Michael B., Mark J. Stern, and Jamie J. Fader. 2005. "The New African American Inequality." *Journal of American History* 92, no. 1: 75–108.

Kevles, Daniel. (1985) 1995. *In the Name of Eugenics: Genetics and the Uses of Human Heredity.* Cambridge, MA: Harvard University Press.

Kim, Annice, Shiriki Kumanyika, Daniel Shive, Uzy Igweatu, and Son-Ho Kim. 2010. "Coverage and Framing of Racial and Ethnic Health Disparities in US Newspapers, 1996–2005." *American Journal of Public Health* 100, suppl. 1: S224–31.

Krieger, Nancy, Jarvis Chen, Brent Coull, Pamela Waterman, and Jason Beckfield. 2013. "The Unique Impact of Abolition of Jim Crow Laws on Reducing Inequities in Infant Death Rates and Implications for Choice of Comparison Groups in Analyzing Societal Determinants of Health." *American Journal of Public Health* 103, no. 12: 2234–44.

Krieger, Nancy, and Stephen Sidney. 1996. "Racial Discrimination and Blood Pressure: The CARDIA Study of Young Black and White Adults." *American Journal of Public Health* 86, no. 10: 1370–78.

Krieger, Nancy, David Williams, and N. E. Moss. 1997. "Measuring Social Class in US Public Health Research: Concepts, Methodologies, and Guidelines." *Annual Review of Sociology* 18: 341–78.

Lacy, Karyn. 2007. *Blue-Chip Black: Race, Class, and Status in the New Black Middle Class*. Berkeley: University of California Press.

Lara, Marielena, Christine Gamboa, M. Iya Kahramanian, Leo Morales, and David Bautista. 2005. "Acculturation and Latino Health in the United States: A Review of the Literature and Its Sociopolitical Context." *Annual Review of Public Health* 26, no. 1: 367–97.

LaViest, Thomas. 1989. "Linking Residential Segregation and the Infant Mortality Race Disparity." *Sociology and Social Research* 73, no. 2: n.p.

Lewontin, Richard. 1972. "The Apportionment of Human Diversity." *Evolutionary Biology* 6: 381–98.

Link, Bruce, and Jo Phelan. 1995. "Social Conditions as Fundamental Causes of Disease." *Journal of Health and Social Behavior* 35, suppl. 1: 80–94.

Lopez, Russ P. 2009. "Public Health, the APHA, and Urban Renewal." *American Journal of Public Health* 99, no. 9: 1603–11.

Lynch, Julia F., and Isabel M. Perera. 2017. "Framing Health Inequity: US Health Disparities in Comparative Perspective." *Journal of Health Politics, Policy and Law* 42, no. 5: 803–39.

McBride, David. 1991. *From TB to AIDS: Epidemics among Urban Blacks since 1900*. Albany: State University of New York Press.

McEwen, Bruce, and Peter Gianaros. 2010. "Central Role of the Brain in Stress and Adaptation: Links to Socioeconomic Status, Health, and Disease." *Annals of the New York Academy of Sciences* 1186, no. 1: 190–222.

Minkler, Meredith, Victoria Vásquez, and Peggy Shepard. 2006. "Promoting Environmental Health Policy through Community-Based Participatory Research: A Case Study from Harlem, New York." *Journal of Urban Health* 83, no. 1: 101–10.

Minkler, Meredith, Victoria Vásquez, Mansoureh Tajik, and Dana Petersen. 2006. "Promoting Environmental Justice through Community-Based Participatory Research: The Role of Community and Partnership Capacity." *Health Behavior and Education* 35, no. 1: 119–37.

Molina, Natalia. 2006. *Fit to Be Citizens? Public Health and Race in Los Angeles, 1879–1939*. Berkeley: University of California Press.

Montagu, Ashley. (1942) 1974. *Man's Most Dangerous Myth: The Fallacy of Race*. New York: Oxford University Press.

Montez, Jennifer, and Anna Zajacova. 2013. "Explaining the Widening Education Gap in Mortality among US White Women." *Journal of Health and Social Behavior* 54, no. 2: 166–82.

Morgan, Edmund. *American Slavery, American Freedom: The Ordeal of Colonial Virginia*. New York: W.W. Norton.

Moynihan, Daniel P. 1965. *The Negro Family: The Case for National Action*. Washington, DC: US Government Printing Office.

Murray, Charles, and Richard Herrnstein. 1994. *The Bell Curve: Intelligence and Class Structure in American Life*. New York: Free Press.

Mustillo, Sarah, Nancy Krieger, Erica Gunderson, Stephen Sidney, Heather McCreath, and Catarina Kiefe. 2004. "Self-Reported Experiences of Racial Discrimination and Black–White Differences in Preterm and Low-Birthweight Deliveries: The CARDIA Study." *American Journal of Public Health* 94, no. 12: 2125–31.

Myrdal, Gunnar. 1944. *An American Dilemma: The Negro Problem and Modern Democracy*. New York: Harper and Row.

Ngai, Mae. 1999. "The Architecture of Race in American Immigration Law: A Reexamination of the Immigration Act of 1924." *Journal of American History* 86, no. 2: 67–92.

O'Connor, Alice. 2001. *Poverty Knowledge: Social Science, Social Policy, and the Poor in Twentieth-Century US History*. Princeton, NJ: Princeton University Press.

Pattillo, Mary. 1999. *Black Picket Fences: Privilege and Peril among the Black Middle Class*. Chicago: University of Chicago Press.

Phillips-Fein, Kim. 2017. *Fear City: New York's Fiscal Crisis and the Rise of Austerity Politics*. New York: W. W. Norton and Company.

Piketty, Thomas. 2013. *Capital in the Twenty-First Century*. Cambridge, MA: Harvard University Press.

Pitts, Steven. 2011. "Research Brief: Black Workers and the Public Sector." UC Berkeley Labor Center, April 4. laborcenter.berkeley.edu/pdf/2011/blacks_public_sector11.pdf.

Rajagopalan, Ramya, and Joan Fujimura. 2012. "Making History via DNA, Making DNA from History: Deconstructing the Race-Disease Connection in Admixture Mapping." In *Genetics and the Unsettled Past: The Collision of DNA, Race, and History*, edited by Keith Wailoo, Alondra Nelson, and Catherine Lee, 143–63. New Brunswick, NJ: Rutgers University Press.

Reed, Adolph. 1997. *W. E. B. Du Bois and American Political Thought: Fabianism and the Color Line*. New York: Oxford University Press.

Reed, Toure. 2008. *Not Alms but Opportunity: The Urban League and the Politics of Racial Uplift, 1910–1950*. Chapel Hill: University of North Carolina Press.

Reverby, Susan. 2009. *Examining Tuskegee: The Infamous Syphilis Study*. Chapel Hill: University of North Carolina Press.

Risch, Neil, Esteban Burchard, Elad Ziv, and Hua Tang. 2002. "Categorization of Humans in Biomedical Research: Genes, Race, and Disease." *Genome Biology* 3, no. 7: 1–12.

Roberts, Samuel. 2009. *Infectious Fear: Politics, Disease, and the Health Effects of Segregation*. Chapel Hill: University of North Carolina Press.

Roux, Ana Diez. 2001. "Investigating Neighborhood and Area Effects on Health." *American Journal of Public Health* 91, no 11: 1783–89.

Schulz, Amy, David Williams, Barbara Israel, and Lora Bex. 2002. "Racial and Spatial Relations as Fundamental Determinants of Health in Detroit." *Milbank Quarterly* 80, no. 4: 677–707.

Self, Robert. 2003. *American Babylon: Race and the Struggle for Postwar Oakland*. Princeton, NJ: Princeton University Press.

Shah, Nayan. 2001. *Contagious Divides: Epidemics and Race in San Francisco's Chinatown*. Berkeley: University of California Press.

Smith, Susan. 1995. *Sick and Tired of Being Sick and Tired: Black Women's Health Activism in America, 1890–1950*. Philadelphia: University of Pennsylvania Press.

Souther, J. Mark. 2017. *Believing in Cleveland: Managing Decline in "The Best Location in the Nation."* Philadelphia: Temple University Press.

Stocking, George W., Jr. 1968. "The Persistence of Polygenist Thought in Post-Darwinian Anthropology." In *Race, Culture, and Evolution: Essays in the History of Anthropology*, 42–68. New York: Free Press.

Sugrue, Thomas. 1996. *Origins of the Urban Crisis: Race and Inequality in Postwar Detroit*. Princeton, NJ: Princeton University Press.

Sze, Julie. 2007. *Noxious New York: The Racial Politics of Urban Health and Environmental Justice*. Cambridge, MA: MIT Press.

Tang, Hua, Tom Quertermous, Beatriz Rodriguez, Sharon L. R. Kardia, Xiaofeng Zhu, Andrew Brown, James S. Pankow, et al. 2005. "Genetic Structure, Self-Identified Race/Ethnicity, and Confounding in Case-Control Association Studies." *American Journal of Human Genetics* 76, no. 2: 268–75.

Thomas, Karen Kruse. 2011. *Deluxe Jim Crow: Civil Rights and American Health Policy, 1935–1954*. Athens: University of Georgia Press.

UNESCO (United Nations Educational, Scientific, and Cultural Organization). 1969. "Statement on Race, Paris, July 1950." In *Four Statements on the Race Question*, 30–36. refugeestudies.org/UNHCR/UNHCR.%20Four%20Statements%20on%20the%20Race%20Question.pdf (accessed October 15, 2021).

Viseltear, Arthur. 1967. *The Watts Hospital: A Health Facility Is Planned for A Metropolitan Slum Area*. Arlington, VA: US Department of Health, Education and Welfare.

Wacquant, Loïc. 2002 "From Slavery to Mass Incarceration: Rethinking the 'Race Question' in the US." *New Left Review*, no. 13: 41–60.

Wacquant, Loïc. 2007. "Territorial Stigmatization in the Age of Advanced Marginality." *Thesis Eleven* 91, no. 1: 66–77.

Williams, David, and Chiquita Collins. 1995. "US Socioeconomic and Racial Differences in Health: Patterns and Explanations." *Annual Review of Sociology* 21: 349–86.

Williams, David, and Chiquita Collins. 2001. "Racial Residential Segregation: A Fundamental Cause of Racial Disparities in Health." *Public Health Reports* 116, no. 5: 404–16.

Williams, David, Jourdyn Lawrence, and Brigette Davis. 2019. "Racism and Health: Evidence and Needed Research." *Annual Review of Public Health* 40: 105–25

Willoughby, Christopher. 2017. "'His Native, Hot Country': Racial Science and Environment in Antebellum American Medical Thought." *Journal of the History of Medicine and Allied Sciences* 72, no. 3: 328–51.

Wilson, William J. 1987. *The Truly Disadvantaged: The Inner City, the Underclass, and Public Policy*. Chicago: University of Chicago Press.

Wolff, Megan. 2006. "The Myth of the Actuary: Life Insurance and Frederick L. Hoffman's *Race Traits and Tendencies of the American Negro*." *Public Health Reports* 121, no. 1: 84–91.

Yudell, Michael. 2014. *Race Unmasked: Biology and Race in the Twentieth Century*. New York: Columbia University Press.

Zuberi, Tukufu. 2003. *Thicker Than Blood: How Racial Statistics Lie*. Minneapolis: University of Minnesota Press.

No Equity without Data Equity: Data Reporting Gaps for Native Hawaiians and Pacific Islanders as Structural Racism

Brittany N. Morey
University of California, Irvine

Richard Calvin Chang
University of Chicago

Karla Blessing Thomas
University of Southern California

'Alisi Tulua
Native Hawaiian and Pacific Islander Data Policy Lab

Corina Penaia
Asian Pacific Islander Forward Movement

Vananh D. Tran
University of California, Los Angeles

Nicholas Pierson
John C. Greer
University of Chicago

Malani Bydalek
University of California, Irvine

Ninez Ponce
University of California, Los Angeles

Abstract Data on the health and social determinants for Native Hawaiians and Pacific Islanders (NHPIs) in the United States are hidden, because data are often not collected or are reported in aggregate with other racial/ethnic groups despite decades of calls to disaggregate NHPI data. As a form of structural racism, data omissions contribute to systemic problems such as inability to advocate, lack of resources, and limitations on political power. The authors conducted a data audit to determine how US federal agencies are collecting and reporting disaggregated NHPI data. Using the COVID-19 pandemic as a case study, they reviewed how states are reporting NHPI cases and deaths. They then used California's neighborhood equity metric—the California

Journal of Health Politics, Policy and Law, Vol. 47, No. 2, April 2022
DOI 10.1215/03616878-9517177

Healthy Places Index (HPI)—to calculate the extent of NHPI underrepresentation in communities targeted for COVID-19 resources in that state. Their analysis shows that while collection and reporting of NHPI data nationally has improved, federal data gaps remain. States are vastly underreporting: more than half of states are not reporting NHPI COVID-19 case and death data. The HPI, used to inform political decisions about allocation of resources to combat COVID-19 in at-risk neighborhoods, underrepresents NHPIs. The authors make recommendations for improving NHPI data equity to achieve health equity and social justice.

Keywords structural racism, Native Hawaiians and Pacific Islanders, data equity, health equity, COVID-19

For decades Native Hawaiian and Pacific Islander (NHPI) leaders in the United States have advocated for disaggregated data that will allow social and health issues to no longer remain invisible in the public eye (Chang, Penaia, and Thomas 2020; Office of Hawaiian Affairs 1982; OMB 1997). NHPIs are diverse, with origins ranging across the Pacific regions of Polynesia, Melanesia, and Micronesia (Hixson, Hepler, and Kim 2012). In the United States, NHPIs account for 0.4% of the population (about 1.4 million people) and are one of the fastest-growing populations (US Census Bureau 2020). Yet data for NHPIs are often hidden as a result of gaps in data collection and reporting (Kana'iaupuni 2011; Panapasa, Crabbe, and Kaholokula 2011; Taualii et al. 2011).[1] The result is that the issues that need attention in NHPI communities are made invisible.

The lack of collected and reported NHPI data equates to a form of structural racism that disproportionately harms NHPI communities (Morey et al. 2020). Structural racism is defined as the ways in which society fosters racial discrimination via macrolevel systems, institutions, ideologies, and processes that result in the reinforcement of discriminatory values, beliefs, and distribution of resources throughout history (Bailey et al. 2017; Gee and Ford 2011). Often supported by interconnected institutions and policies, structural racism does not need to be initiated by a particular individual or group of individuals with racist intent. Rather, structural racism can result from subconscious or automatic disparate treatment that results in harm to historically oppressed people of color (Reskin 2012). Historical and continued oppression of NHPIs can be attributed to settler colonialism—the occupation of Indigenous lands by a society of settlers through the forcible

1. Data may be collected improperly in surveys that do not provide a separate race category for NHPI identification on forms. Data may be reported improperly by aggregating NHPIs with Asians or other race categories prior to releasing the data.

removal of Indigenous peoples—which results in the continued erasure of these populations in public discourse (Tuck and Yang 2012).

Structural racism and settler colonialism manifest to harm NHPI communities through data gaps and limitations. With limited data on health disparities, public health efforts to support NHPI health are underresourced (Samoa et al. 2020). NHPI policy advocates experience decreased political power because of lack of data on social and health inequities, limiting their ability to advocate for policy changes (Morey et al. 2020). The complete omission of NHPI data or aggregation of it with other racial groups, often with Asian Americans, reinforces the marginalization that NHPIs experience in US society (Chang, Penaia, and Thomas 2020; Kaholokula et al. 2020). In this article, we contend that social and health equity for NHPIs can be achieved when there is equity in the collection and reporting of data, especially in conjunction with community-based mobilization of health-promoting measures informed by those data.

Background

On October 30, 1997, the OMB announced revisions to the standards for the classification of federal data on race and ethnicity (OMB 1997). This notice, which revised the initial classifications provided by Statistical Policy Directive Number 15 (also known as OMB 15), created 30 years prior, included three major modifications: (1) treating the Asian or Pacific Islander category as two separate categories—"Asian" and "Native Hawaiian or Other Pacific Islander," (2) changing the term "Hispanic" to "Hispanic or Latino," and (3) allowing more than one self-identified race.[2] The implementation of these revisions represented a major milestone for those identifying as Native Hawaiian or Other Pacific Islander, reflecting hard-fought efforts to advocate for changes to the standard race classifications that previously aggregated Asians and Pacific Islanders together.[3]

The aggregation of NHPIs with Asians rendered NHPI health and social inequities invisible, because Asians represent a significantly larger population that is more socioeconomically advantaged on average

2. Allowing people to self-identify with more than one race on forms, rather than automatically having people mark a single "multiracial" category, helps with identifying the diversity of multiracial people. This is important for NHPIs, more than half of whom are multiracial but who often strongly identify with their NHPI ancestry, as described below.

3. Historically, NHPIs have often been aggregated with Asians to increase political and social influence, achieving common goals as a broad panethnic group (see Okamoto and Mora 2014). However, automatically using the "Asian and Pacific Islander" panethnic category beyond the purpose of these efforts has also inflicted harm on the relatively smaller NHPI grouping (see Tuck and Yang 2012).

(Kana'iaupuni 2011; Panapasa, Crabbe, and Kaholokula 2011; Taualii et al. 2011). Compared to Asian American populations as an aggregate group, NHPI populations experience higher rates of chronic and infectious disease and have very different profiles regarding the social determinants of health leading to such health inequities, including lower educational attainment, higher rates of poverty, and limited access to preventive health care (Hixson, Hepler, and Kim 2012; US Census Bureau 2020). Disaggregating NHPIs from Asians acknowledges these experiences, which also reflect differences in the histories, cultures, languages, and ancestries of these groups (Hosaka, Castanera, and Yamada 2021).[4] The OMB's racial and ethnic categories are important because they set the minimum standard for federal data on the classification of race/ethnicity used to produce demographic data as well as to monitor civil rights enforcement and inform program implementation.

The revisions to the OMB 15 race and ethnic classification standards in 1997 did not arise automatically. The process began in 1993, when the OMB underwent a comprehensive review of the categories used to measure race and ethnicity (OMB 1997). This occurred after the OMB received criticism following the 1990 US Census from members of the public who felt that the minimum categories inadequately reflected the diversity of the nation's population. The comprehensive review of the OMB racial/ethnic classifications included hearings, testimony, and a research agenda by the Interagency Committee to evaluate the effect of possible changes to the racial and ethnic categories. In 1997, the OMB released a *Federal Register* notice (62 FR 36874—36946) requesting public comment on the Interagency Committee's Report to the OMB on the Review of Statistical Policy Directive No. 15.

However, the Interagency Committee recommended that data on Native Hawaiians continue to be classified in the "Asian or Pacific Islander" category. In response, the OMB received approximately 300 letters and 7,000 individually signed and mailed preprinted yellow postcards specifically on the issue of classifying Native Hawaiian data separately from Asians. The OMB additionally received about 500 signed form letters from members of the Hapa[5] Issues Forum in support of reporting multiple races. More than half of NHPIs identify as multiracial (Hixson, Hepler, and Kim

4. Although it is important to note that the OMB racial/ethnic standards for classification make it clear that these categories do not reflect scientific (i.e., biological or genetic) or anthropometric (i.e., phenotypic) distinctions, these categories may reflect social characteristics placed in the context of the experiences and histories of these groups (OMB 1997).

5. *Hapa* is a Hawaiian word that traditionally refers to someone of mixed Native Hawaiian and foreign ancestry.

2012; US Census Bureau 2020). The 7,000 individuals who signed and sent preprinted yellow postcards, the Hawaiian congressional delegation, the departments and legislature of the government of the state of Hawaiʻi, Hawaiian organizations, and individual advocates strongly opposed the Interagency Committee's recommendation. Their arguments supported reclassifying Native Hawaiians with American Indians or Alaska Natives, given their identification as the original inhabitants of Hawaiʻi. Their comments further expressed that disaggregated data were needed to monitor the socioeconomic conditions of Native Hawaiians and to address systematic discrimination against this population in housing, education, employment, and other sectors. At the time, Native Hawaiian advocates did not request a separate category for Native Hawaiians, because the Interagency Committee had expressed opposition to adding more race categories to the original four OMB 15 race categories (American Indian or Alaska Native, Asian or Pacific Islander, Black, and white). In the end, the OMB decided to add the fifth category, splitting the "Asian or Pacific Islander" category into two: "Asian" and "Native Hawaiian or Other Pacific Islander." The latter was defined as a "person having origins in any of the original peoples of Hawaiʻi, Guam, Sāmoa, or other Pacific Islands." At the time, it was estimated that about 60% of the NHPI category would consist of Native Hawaiians, but it would also include Carolinians, Fijians, Guamanians (Chamorros), Kosraeans, Melanesians, Micronesians, Northern Mariana Islanders, Palauans, Papua New Guineans, Ponapeans (Pohnpelans), Polynesians, Sāmoans, Solomon Islanders, Tahitians, Tarawa Islanders, Tokelauans, Tongans, Trukese (Chuukese), and Yapese. The revised race and ethnicity OMB standards reflect a federal review process that was shaped by the urgent desires of NHPI community members and organizations.

By treating NHPIs as a separate race category, the 1997 revised OMB 15 standards allowed for greater attention to be paid to the health, social, and economic issues that would affect NHPI populations in the future. The important implications of this disaggregation of NHPIs from the "Asian Pacific Islander" category become apparent in times of crisis, including during the COVID-19 pandemic. Initial COVID-19 disaggregated data in the states of Arkansas, California, Colorado, Hawaiʻi, Oregon, Utah, and Washington (some of the first states to report COVID-19 data by race for NHPIs) in the spring of 2020 revealed that NHPIs were experiencing the highest rates of COVID-19 cases and deaths of any other racial/ethnic group in those states (Chang, Penaia, and Thomas 2020). These early reports led a coalition of NHPI community leaders to form the National Pacific Islander

COVID-19 Response Team (NPICRT) (Samoa et al. 2020). The NPICRT championed the formation of the NHPI Data Policy Lab—housed at the UCLA Center for Health Policy Research—comprising researchers, data analysts, and policy advocates who would consolidate and represent NHPI data to inform COVID-19 advocacy efforts from the local to the national levels. However, as members of the NHPI Data Policy Lab quickly learned, there was and continues to be inconsistent collection and reporting of NHPI COVID-19 case and death data across states and localities, obstructing grassroots efforts to respond to NHPI community needs in those areas during the pandemic (Chang, Penaia, and Thomas 2020).

Given this context, an up-to-date review of compliance with the 1997 revised OMB 15 standards is warranted. In 2011, Panapasa, Crabbe, and Kaholokula (2011) reviewed data sources from federal agencies for compliance with the 1997 revised OMB 15 standard on the collection and reporting of NHPI data. They found that while these data sources were collecting disaggregated NHPI data appropriately, the vast majority of the data sources were not reporting NHPI data. Panapasa, Crabbe, and Kaholokula highlighted the ongoing problems with data reporting for NHPIs that are the result of inadequate sample sizes or inappropriate reaggregation of NHPIs into "Asian American or Pacific Islander" or "Other race" groups. The authors made recommendations to increase efforts to oversample NHPI populations, create reliable data estimates, and partner with NHPI communities in federal data sources. Nevertheless, special surveillance efforts are often needed. An example is the 2014 NHPI National Health Interview Survey (NHPI NHIS), the first and largest nationally representative survey of NHPI health conducted by the Center for Disease Control and Prevention's National Center for Health Statistics (National Center for Health Statistics 2014).[6]

NHPIs continue to be systematically missed in efforts to achieve health equity (Morey et al. 2020). In recent years, more attention has been given to issues of neighborhood inequity, including environmental injustices that are the result of the overlapping issues of residential segregation, concentrated poverty, decreased political power, disproportionate pollution burden, poor health infrastructure, lack of green space, unsafe built environments, and more (Diez Roux and Mair 2010; Pastor and Morello-Frosch 2014). While these are important issues, NHPIs have often been excluded

6. Although the NHPI NHIS is nationally representative and the first of its kind, it is a standalone cross-sectional survey and is not incorporated into the National Health Interview Survey.

from efforts that mitigate neighborhood injustices (Morey 2014). It is more common now to rely on indices that calculate neighborhood social disadvantage and disease risk in plans for the distribution of limited resources (Maizlish et al. 2019). Unfortunately, NHPI community members report that these neighborhood measures often miss NHPI populations. Therefore, policies that rely on these widely used neighborhood indices may systematically exclude NHPIs—another example of structural racism.

In the current study, we assess data equity for NHPIs as structural racism in three ways. First, we reassess the federal data sources reviewed by Panapasa, Crabbe, and Kaholokula (2011) 10 years ago for compliance with the revised OMB 15 standards for collecting and reporting NHPI data, adding some additional data sources that are relevant for understanding health and social determinants of health for NHPI populations nationally. Second, using the COVID-19 pandemic as a case study, we review the public availability of NHPI case and death data for COVID-19 by state. Third, we evaluate within the state of California the use of a health equity metric—the California Healthy Places Index—as an indicator of neighborhood disadvantage, to determine whether NHPIs and other communities of color are underrepresented in "high risk" neighborhoods. The goal of these three steps is to demonstrate how data inequity operates on a national, state, and local level, with implications for health equity and social justice efforts for NHPI populations.

Methods

Review of Federal Data Sources' Collection and Reporting of NHPI Data

In the first analysis, we reviewed national data based on those datasets first reviewed by Panapasa, Crabbe, and Kaholokula (2011) to determine progress in the past 10 years on the collection and/or reporting of NHPI data. The 2011 paper originally reviewed data from six federal agencies: the Department of Commerce, the Department of Health and Human Services, the Department of Education, the Department of Agriculture, the Department of Housing and Urban Development, and the Department of Justice. We reviewed 19 of the original 20 data sources.[7] In addition, we selected 10 other national datasets to review, based on the criteria originally used to select datasets: (1) accessibility, (2) degree of national

7. One data source—the National Hospital Discharge Survey—was not included because data collection is no longer ongoing.

coverage of the US population, and (3) potential source of information for policy and intervention. We added a fourth criterion: collection of data is current and ongoing. In total, we reviewed 29 national datasets. The data sources are not an exhaustive list, but they represent datasets that collect and report race/ethnicity that could be useful for informing future policy decisions or to conduct research illuminating health disparities and their underlying social determinants. For each data source, we examined the public websites to determine whether NHPI data were being collected and reported, and if so, how these data were being collected and reported.[8] At least two authors examined the public websites for each data source for evidence (i.e., text descriptions of available data, links to datasets, data outputs, codebooks, questionnaires, etc.) of how data on race was being collected and reported in the survey. This allowed us to determine compliance with the revised OMB 15 standards and to assess the level of disaggregation of NHPI data. We also made note of whether NHPI data collection or reporting had changed from 2011 to 2021 in the data sources previously reviewed.

Review of NHPI US COVID-19 Case and Death Data in States

To assess COVID-19 data in states, we used data from the NHPI COVID-19 Data Policy Lab Dashboard (UCLA Center for Health Policy Research 2021). This dashboard systematically reports NHPI COVID-19 case and death rates in states that disaggregate NHPI data. The dashboard collected counts of COVID-19 cases and deaths from the COVID Tracking Project and the Hawai'i COVID-19 Dashboard, and it calculated rates using American Community Survey 2015–2019 five-year population estimates ("The Covid Tracking Project" 2021; Hawai'i Department of Health 2021; US Census Bureau 2020). Of states that do not report disaggregated NHPI data, the dashboard provides information on how NHPI data are being treated in those states. We used these data to calculate the number and percentage of states in each of these categories separately for COVID-19 cases and deaths: (1) reports disaggregated NHPI data, (2) uses the obsolete panracial "Asian Pacific Islander" category, (3) specifies NHPI data under the "Other race" category, (4) does not specify an NHPI reporting practice, (5) does not report any race/ethnicity data, or (6) does not disaggregate NHPI death data (for COVID-19 death rates only). Data were up to date as of February 21, 2021.

8. Most surveys determine race/ethnicity by self-report, which is preferable and likely most accurate. Other data sources (e.g., death certificate data) use the report of a proxy (e.g., coroner or doctor) and may have lower accuracy.

Evaluation of the California Healthy Places Index in Representing NHPIs in California Census Tracts

On August 28, 2020, California Governor Gavin Newsom announced the "Blueprint for a Safer Economy," which included a health equity metric—the California Healthy Places Index (HPI)—that would be used to determine which counties could move to less restrictive reopening tiers.[9] The stated purpose of applying the health equity metric was to incentivize a reduction in disease transmission for all communities, especially those disproportionately impacted by COVID-19. We downloaded HPI data for California census tracts from the Public Health Alliance of Southern California's website (Public Health Alliance of Southern California 2021). The HPI provides an index score for all 2010 California census tracts with a population of 1,500 or more. The HPI includes 25 different community characteristics combined into a single score at various geographic levels. The 25 characteristics fall into eight policy action domains, including economic (e.g., income), social (e.g., two-parent households), education (e.g., bachelor's degree or higher), transportation (e.g., automobile access), built environment (e.g., park access), housing (e.g., homeownership), clean environment (e.g., ozone), and health care (e.g., insured). Notably, the HPI does not include measures of race or ethnicity to allow state agencies to remain compliant with California Proposition 209, which prohibits the use of race or ethnicity for allocating public resources.[10] Each included domain was weighted, contributing to an overall HPI score. Based on the distribution of the HPI score across California census tracts, the HPI places census tracts into four numbered quartiles of neighborhood disadvantage, with quartile 4 indicating the highest level of neighborhood disadvantage (i.e., bottom quartile). These quartiles are used to make public policy decisions about which neighborhoods are most disadvantaged, with the bottom-quartile neighborhoods representing those that may be identified for additional resources during public health emergencies.

9. The HPI health equity metric applied to California counties with more than 106,000 residents. For a county to move to a less restrictive tier, it must meet specific COVID-19 case and test positivity rates within their lowest-quartile HPI (i.e., most disadvantaged) census tracts. The Blueprint for a Safer Economy: Equity Focus can be found at www.cdph.ca.gov/Programs/CID/DCDC/Pages/COVID-19/CaliforniaHealthEquityMetric.aspx.

10. Proposition 209, approved by voters in 1996, is a constitutional amendment that reads: "The State cannot discriminate against or grant preferential treatment on the basis of race, sex, color, ethnicity or national origin in the operation of public employment, public education, and public contracting" (California Constitution article I, section 31). This amendment essentially bans the use of race/ethnicity or nationality as the basis of appropriating state resources, including resources to combat COVID-19.

We then determined whether racial/ethnic groups are underrepresented in these most disadvantaged neighborhoods as defined by the HPI. We used American Community Survey 2015–2019 5-year data to determine the population of each of six OMB single racial/ethnic groups (Hispanic/Latino, white, Black, American Indian/Alaska Native, Asian, or NHPI) in counties and census tracts (US Census Bureau 2020). To determine whether the HPI underrepresented each racial/ethnic group, we calculated whether the total percentage of the racial/ethnic group residing within bottom-quartile (most disadvantaged) census tracts in a county according to the HPI was lower than the percentage of the racial/ethnic group in the county's total population. Using this standard, of the total 43 counties in California with census tract level HPI, we identified the number of counties where each racial/ethnic group is underrepresented by the HPI in bottom-quartile census tracts. We then calculated the percentage of counties that underrepresent that group by dividing the number of counties by 43 and multiplying by 100. We listed the California counties with a population greater than 150,000 where the HPI underrepresents communities of color in bottom-quartile census tracts (29 of the total 43 California counties have populations greater than150,000). Underrepresentation was conceptualized this way since the California Blueprint for a Safer Economy would likely incentivize resources for these census tracts in the lowest HPI quartile. However, it was unclear whether these resources would help NHPI communities or underrepresent them despite these communities having the highest statewide COVID-19 case rates of any racial/ethnic group.

Results

Review of Federal Collection and Reporting of NHPI Data

Table 1 displays the results of our review of 29 sources of federal data for compliance with the 1997 revised OMB 15 standards for collecting and reporting NHPI data. Of the 29 federal data sources, the majority (26, or 90%) are collecting data for NHPIs as a separate race category. The three data sources that are not in compliance with the revised OMB 15 standards are either collecting data inconsistently by state, are erroneously collecting data using the panracial Asian or Pacific Islander category, or are no longer collecting race data. Of the 29 federal data sources, 19 (66%) are reporting data for NHPIs as a separate race category. When data for NHPIs are not being reported separately, it is usually the result of NHPI data being

Table 1 Review of Federal Data Sources for Compliance with Revised OMB 15 Guidelines for Reporting Disaggregated Native Hawaiian and Pacific Islander (NHPI) Data

Federal agency and data source	Collecting data using OMB 15? (yes/no)	How are data collected for NHPIs? (racial/ethnic categories)	Reporting data for NHPIs using OMB 15? (yes/no)	How are data reported for NHPIs? (racial/ethnic categories, aggregated, other race, or NHPI subgroup)	Change in data collection or reporting since Panapasa, Crabbe, and Kaholokula (2011) review
1. Department of Commerce					
US Census FY 2000, 2010, 2020	Yes	Detailed NHPI race	Yes	NHPI total, alone or in combination, Polynesian, Micronesian, or Melanesian, Native Hawaiian, Sāmoan, Tongan, other Polynesian, Guamanian or Chamorro, Marshallese, other Micronesian, Fijian, other Melanesian, other Pacific Islander (not specified)	No; compliant

(*continued*)

Table 1 Review of Federal Data Sources for Compliance with Revised OMB 15 Guidelines for Reporting Disaggregated Native Hawaiian and Pacific Islander (NHPI) Data *(continued)*

Federal agency and data source	Collecting data using OMB 15? (yes/no)	How are data collected for NHPIs? (racial/ethnic categories)	Reporting data for NHPIs using OMB 15? (yes/no)	How are data reported for NHPIs? (racial/ethnic categories, aggregated, other race, or NHPI subgroup)	Change in data collection or reporting since Panapasa, Crabbe, and Kaholokula (2011) review
American Community Survey (multiple years)	Yes	Detailed NHPI race	Yes	NHPI alone or in combination, Native Hawaiian, Guamanian or Chamorro, other Micronesian, Sāmoan, Tongan, Fijian, other Pacific Islander (not specified)	Yes; improvement in reporting
Current Population Survey	Yes	NHPI, Native Hawaiian, Guamanian or Chamorro, Sāmoan, other Pacific Islander	Yes	NHPI alone, NHPI alone or in combination	Yes; improvement in reporting

Table 1 *(continued)*

Federal agency and data source	Collecting data using OMB 15? (yes/no)	How are data collected for NHPIs? (racial/ethnic categories)	Reporting data for NHPIs using OMB 15? (yes/no)	How are data reported for NHPIs? (racial/ethnic categories, aggregated, other race, or NHPI subgroup)	Change in data collection or reporting since Panapasa, Crabbe, and Kaholokula (2011) review
Survey of Income and Program Participation	Yes	NHPI	Yes	Native Hawaiian or other Pacific Islander alone, white-NHPI, Black-NHPI, Asian-NHPI, white-Asian-NHPI, other 4 or more races	Not included in previous review
2. Department of Health and Human Services					
National Vital Statistics System	Yes	Detailed NHPI race	Partial*	For births: NHPI alone, NHPI in combination; for deaths: Hawaiian (includes multiracial), other Asian or Pacific Islander	No; reporting noncompliant
National Longitudinal Mortality Study	Yes	Detailed NHPI race	Yes	NHPI alone, NHPI in combination, Hawaiian, other Pacific Islander (e.g., Sāmoan, Guamanian, Tongan)	No; compliant

(continued)

Table 1 Review of Federal Data Sources for Compliance with Revised OMB 15 Guidelines for Reporting Disaggregated Native Hawaiian and Pacific Islander (NHPI) Data *(continued)*

Federal agency and data source	Collecting data using OMB 15? (yes/no)	How are data collected for NHPIs? (racial/ethnic categories)	Reporting data for NHPIs using OMB 15? (yes/no)	How are data reported for NHPIs? (racial/ethnic categories, aggregated, other race, or NHPI subgroup)	Change in data collection or reporting since Panapasa, Crabbe, and Kaholokula (2011) review
National Health Interview Survey	Yes	Native Hawaiian, other Pacific Islander	No	For public data: other single and multiple races, Non-Hispanic Asian Indian or Alaska Native and any other group; for restricted data: non-Hispanic NHPI only, non-Hispanic other only, all other combinations	No; reporting noncompliant
National Health and Nutrition Examination Survey	Yes	Native Hawaiian or Pacific Islander and specific subgroup: Native Hawaiian, Guamanian/Chamorro, Sāmoan, other Pacific Islander	No	Other race including multiracial	No; reporting noncompliant

Table 1 *(continued)*

Federal agency and data source	Collecting data using OMB 15? (yes/no)	How are data collected for NHPIs? (racial/ethnic categories)	Reporting data for NHPIs using OMB 15? (yes/no)	How are data reported for NHPIs? (racial/ethnic categories, aggregated, other race, or NHPI subgroup)	Change in data collection or reporting since Panapasa, Crabbe, and Kaholokula (2011) review
National Survey of Family Growth	Yes	Respondent's race: Native Hawaiian, Guamanian or Chamorro, Sāmoan, other Pacific Islander; child and spouse race: Native Hawaiian or other Pacific Islander	No	Other race	No; reporting noncompliant
Behavioral Risk Factor Surveillance System	Yes	Pacific Islander and subcategories: Native Hawaiian, Guamanian, Chamorro, Sāmoan, other Pacific Islander	Yes	NHPI only, multiracial	Yes; improvement in reporting

(continued)

Table 1 Review of Federal Data Sources for Compliance with Revised OMB 15 Guidelines for Reporting Disaggregated Native Hawaiian and Pacific Islander (NHPI) Data (*continued*)

Federal agency and data source	Collecting data using OMB 15? (yes/no)	How are data collected for NHPIs? (racial/ethnic categories)	Reporting data for NHPIs using OMB 15? (yes/no)	How are data reported for NHPIs? (racial/ethnic categories, aggregated, other race, or NHPI subgroup)	Change in data collection or reporting since Panapasa, Crabbe, and Kaholokula (2011) review
National Hospital Ambulatory Medical Care Survey	Yes	Native Hawaiian or other Pacific Islander	No	Unknown	No; reporting noncompliant
National Survey on Drug Use and Health	Yes	Native Hawaiian, Guamanian or Chamorro, Sāmoan, other Pacific Islander	Yes	Native Hawaiian or other Pacific Islander	Yes; improvement in reporting
Medical Expenditure Panel Survey	Yes	Native Hawaiian, Guamanian or Chamorro, Sāmoan, other Pacific Islander	No	Asian/Native Hawaiian/other Pacific Islander	No; reporting noncompliant
Youth Risk Behavior Surveillance System	Yes	Native Hawaiian or other Pacific Islander	Yes	Non-Hispanic Native Hawaiian/other Pacific Islander race only (does not include multiracial)	Not included in previous reporting

Table 1 *(continued)*

Federal agency and data source	Collecting data using OMB 15? (yes/no)	How are data collected for NHPIs? (racial/ethnic categories)	Reporting data for NHPIs using OMB 15? (yes/no)	How are data reported for NHPIs? (racial/ethnic categories, aggregated, other race, or NHPI subgroup)	Change in data collection or reporting since Panapasa, Crabbe, and Kaholokula (2011) review
Substance Abuse and Mental Health Services Administration—Mental Health Client-Level Data	Partial depending on state; yes for some, no for others (does not specify specific states)	Native Hawaiian or other Pacific Islander; Asian or Pacific Islander (temporary code)	Yes	Native Hawaiian or other Pacific Islander	Not included in previous reporting
National HIV Behavioral Surveillance	Yes	Native Hawaiian or other Pacific Islander	Yes	Native Hawaiian/other Pacific Islander	Not included in previous reporting
Web-based Injury Statistics Query and Reporting System	No	Asian/Pacific Islander	No	Asian/Pacific Islander	Not included in previous reporting

(continued)

Table 1 Review of Federal Data Sources for Compliance with Revised OMB 15 Guidelines for Reporting Disaggregated Native Hawaiian and Pacific Islander (NHPI) Data *(continued)*

Federal agency and data source	Collecting data using OMB 15? (yes/no)	How are data collected for NHPIs? (racial/ethnic categories)	Reporting data for NHPIs using OMB 15? (yes/no)	How are data reported for NHPIs? (racial/ethnic categories, aggregated, other race, or NHPI subgroup)	Change in data collection or reporting since Panapasa, Crabbe, and Kaholokula (2011) review
3. Department of Education					
Early Childhood Longitudinal Survey	Yes	Detailed NHPI race	No	Non-Hispanic Asian, Hawaiian, or Pacific Islander	Not included in previous reporting
Kindergarten Cohort, Kindergarten Class of 1998–99	Yes	Native Hawaiian or other Pacific Islander	Yes	Non-Hispanic Native Hawaiian/other Pacific Islander race	Yes; improvement in reporting
National Household Education Surveys	Yes	Native Hawaiian or other Pacific Islander	Yes	Native Hawaiian or other Pacific Islander	Yes; improvement in reporting
School Survey on Crime and Safety	No		No		Yes; decrease in reporting; is no longer collecting or reporting race data
Civil Rights Data Collection	Yes	Native Hawaiian or other Pacific Islander	Yes	Native Hawaiian or other Pacific Islander	Not included in previous reporting

Table 1 *(continued)*

Federal agency and data source	Collecting data using OMB 15? (yes/no)	How are data collected for NHPIs? (racial/ ethnic categories)	Reporting data for NHPIs using OMB 15? (yes/no)	How are data reported for NHPIs? (racial/ethnic categories, aggregated, other race, or NHPI subgroup)	Change in data collection or reporting since Panapasa, Crabbe, and Kaholokula (2011) review
National Assessment of Educational Progress	Yes	Native Hawaiian or other Pacific Islander	Yes	Native Hawaiian/other Pacific Islander	Not included in previous reporting
EDFacts	Yes	Native Hawaiian/ other Pacific Islander or Pacific Islander	No	Asian/Pacific Islander	Not included in previous reporting
4. Department of Agriculture					
Supplemental Nutrition Assistance Program Quality Control Database	Yes	Native Hawaiian or other Pacific Islander	Yes	Native Hawaiian or other Pacific Islander	Yes; improvement in reporting
Women, Infants, and Children Program	Yes	Hawaiian/Pacific Islanders	Yes	Hawaiian/Pacific Islanders	Not included in previous reporting

(continued)

Table 1 Review of Federal Data Sources for Compliance with Revised OMB 15 Guidelines for Reporting Disaggregated Native Hawaiian and Pacific Islander (NHPI) Data (*continued*)

Federal agency and data source	Collecting data using OMB 15? (yes/no)	How are data collected for NHPIs? (racial/ethnic categories)	Reporting data for NHPIs using OMB 15? (yes/no)	How are data reported for NHPIs? (racial/ethnic categories, aggregated, other race, or NHPI subgroup)	Change in data collection or reporting since Panapasa, Crabbe, and Kaholokula (2011) review
5. Department of Housing and Urban Development					
American Housing Survey	Yes	Native Hawaiian only, Guamanian or Chamorro only, Sāmoan only, some other Pacific Islander race only, two or more Native Hawaiian or Pacific Islander races, Hawaiian and Pacific Islander only, NHPI mixed with other races	Yes	Native Hawaiian only, Guamanian or Chamorro only, Sāmoan only, some other Pacific Islander race only, two or more Native Hawaiian or Pacific Islander races, Hawaiian and Pacific Islander only, NHPI mixed with other races	Yes; improvement in reporting

Table 1 *(continued)*

Federal agency and data source	Collecting data using OMB 15? (yes/no)	How are data collected for NHPIs? (racial/ethnic categories)	Reporting data for NHPIs using OMB 15? (yes/no)	How are data reported for NHPIs? (racial/ethnic categories, aggregated, other race, or NHPI subgroup)	Change in data collection or reporting since Panapasa, Crabbe, and Kaholokula (2011) review
6. Department of Justice					
Census of Jails	Yes	Native Hawaiian Pacific Islander (non-Hispanic)	Yes	Native Hawaiian or Pacific Islander	No; compliant
National Crime Victimization Survey	Yes	Native Hawaiian or other Pacific Islander	Yes	Native Hawaiian/other Pacific Islander alone, NHPI in combination with one other race	Yes; improvement in reporting

* Data for births are more complete than data for deaths. Completeness and validity of death data vary by state. For deaths, Native Hawaiians are disaggregated, but other Asians are aggregated with Pacific Islanders.

** Disaggregated data are available in restricted data.

Notes: National Hospital Discharge Survey was originally included and reviewed by Panapasa, Crabbe, and Kaholokula (2011) but is not reviewed here because data collection is no longer ongoing.

reported in aggregate with the Asian race category or "other" race category, or it is unclear how NHPI data are being treated.

There was an improvement in the reporting of NHPI data from 2011 to 2021. Of the 19 data sources originally reviewed by Panapasa, Krabbe, and Kaholokula (2011), nine (47%) improved their data-reporting practices and now report NHPI data as a separate race category. In some of these cases, the public data are available but require some downloading of public-use data files and statistical software to access the NHPI data. On the other hand, 6 of the 19 originally reviewed data sources (32%) fail to provide disaggregated NHPI data 10 years later.

Review of State Reporting of NHPI COVID-19 Cases and Deaths

Figure 1 presents maps created by the NHPI COVID-19 Data Policy Lab Dashboard, showing US COVID-19 NHPI cases and deaths by state. As of February 21, 2021, there were 52,695 reported NHPI cases (Figure 1A) and 798 reported NHPI deaths (Figure 1B) in the United States. At that time, the states with the highest NHPI case rates were Louisiana, Alaska, Iowa, Illinois, Idaho, and Minnesota. The states with highest NHPI death rates were Louisiana, Iowa, Illinois, Arkansas, California, and Minnesota.

Table 2 shows that of the 50 states, only 20 (40%) are reporting disaggregated NHPI case data, and only 16 (32%) are reporting disaggregated NHPI death data. Of those not reporting disaggregated NHPI case and death data, nine states (18%) are using the obsolete panracial "Asian Pacific Islander" category, while five states (10%) are including NHPI data in the "other race" category. For the remaining states, it is unclear how NHPI data are being treated, or the states are not reporting COVID-19 data for NHPIs or by race/ethnicity at all. Of the states that are properly reporting disaggregated data, the NHPI rates per 100,000 population rank the highest of any racial group in 16 of 20 (80%) for COVID-19 cases and 11 of 16 (69%) for COVID-19 deaths.

Evaluation of the HPI in Representing NHPIs in California

Table 3 shows for each OMB racial/ethnic group the number and percentage of the 43 California counties where that group is considered underrepresented in the most disadvantaged (4th quartile) census tracts according to the HPI. Results show that the HPI underrepresented certain populations by race in California counties. Of communities of color, Asian Americans were most affected, with 34 (79%) of 43 counties

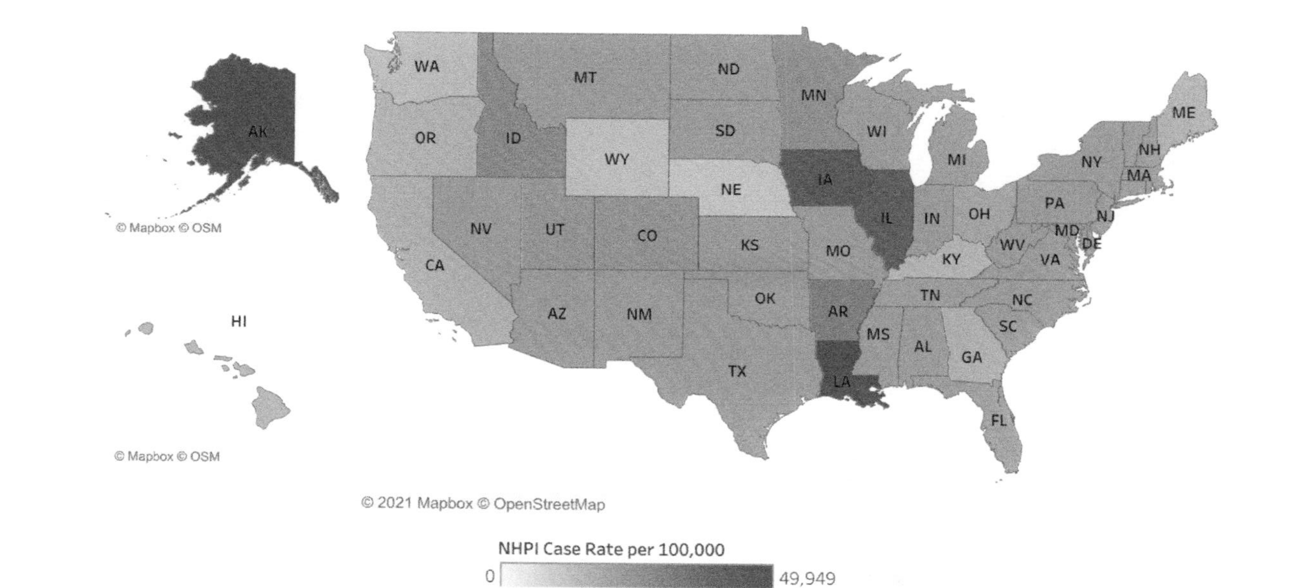

Figure 1 Snapshots of the NHPI Data Policy Lab Dashboard showing COVID-19 case rates and death rates in states reporting disaggregated NHPI data. A. NHPI COVID-19 case rates in states. B. NHPI COVID-19 death rates in states.

Notes: As of February 21, 2021; total NHPI COVID-19 cases: 52,695; total NHPI COVID-19 deaths: 798.

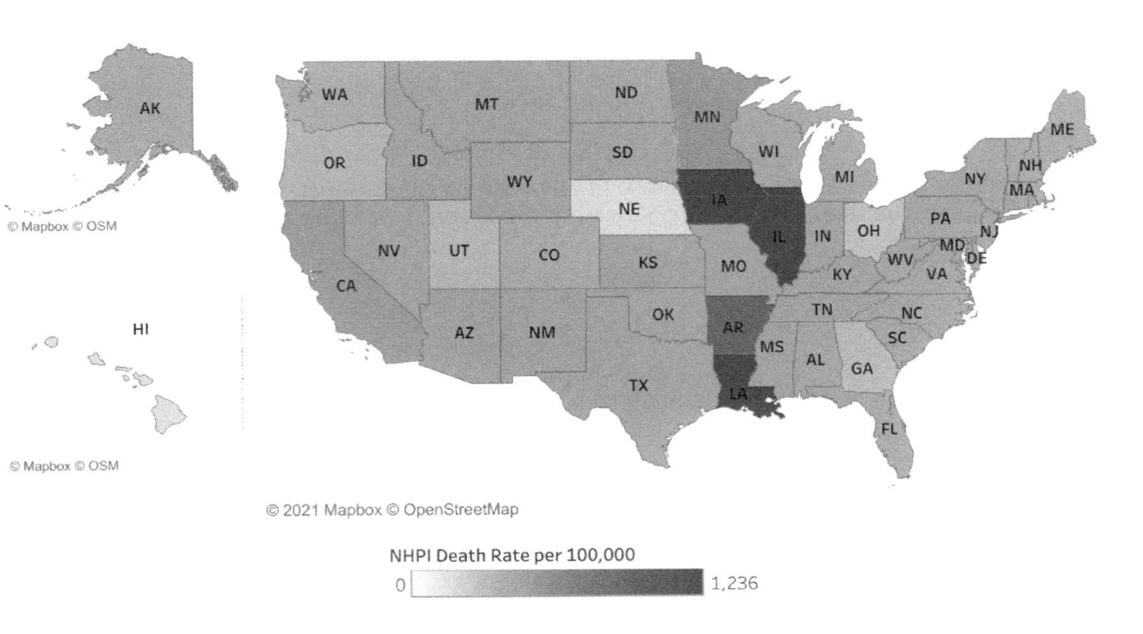

Figure 1 *(continued)*

Table 2 State Reporting Practice of COVID-19 Case and Death Data for NHPI Populations

State	COVID-19 cases					COVID-19 deaths					
	Reporting disaggregated NHPI data	Uses obsolete panracial "Asian Pacific Islander" category	Specifies NHPI data under "other" race category	Does not specify NHPI reporting practice	Does not report any race/ ethnicity data	Reporting disaggregated NHPI data	Uses obsolete panracial "Asian Pacific Islander" category	Specifies NHPI data under "other" race category	Does not specify NHPI reporting practice	Does not report any race/ ethnicity data	Does not report disaggregated NHPI death data
Alabama				x					x		
Alaska	x					x					
Arizona		x					x				
Arkansas	x					x					
California	x					x					
Colorado	x					x					
Connecticut		x					x				
Delaware		x					x				
Florida			x					x			
Georgia	x					x					
Hawaii	x					x					
Idaho	x										x
Illinois	x					x					
Indiana			x					x			
Iowa	x					x					

(continued)

Table 2 State Reporting Practice of COVID-19 Case and Death Data for NHPI Populations *(continued)*

	COVID-19 cases					COVID-19 deaths					
State	Reporting disaggregated NHPI data	Uses obsolete panracial "Asian Pacific Islander" category	Specifies NHPI data under "other" race category	Does not specify NHPI reporting practice	Does not report any race/ethnicity data	Reporting disaggregated NHPI data	Uses obsolete panracial "Asian Pacific Islander" category	Specifies NHPI data under "other" race category	Does not specify NHPI reporting practice	Does not report any race/ethnicity data	Does not report disaggregated NHPI death data
Kansas				x					x		
Kentucky	x										x
Louisiana	x					x					
Maine	x										x
Maryland				x					x		
Massachusetts				x					x		
Michigan		x					x				
Minnesota	x					x					
Mississippi				x					x		
Missouri			x					x			
Montana				x					x		
Nebraska	x					x					
Nevada				x					x		
New Hampshire			x					x			
New Jersey			x					x			

Table 2 *(continued)*

State	COVID-19 cases					COVID-19 deaths					
	Reporting disaggregated NHPI data	Uses obsolete panracial "Asian Pacific Islander" category	Specifies NHPI data under "other" race category	Does not specify NHPI reporting practice	Does not report any race/ ethnicity data	Reporting disaggregated NHPI data	Uses obsolete panracial "Asian Pacific Islander" category	Specifies NHPI data under "other" race category	Does not specify NHPI reporting practice	Does not report any race/ ethnicity data	Does not report disaggregated NHPI death data
New Mexico				x							x
New York		x					x				
North Carolina	x					x					
North Dakota					x					x	
Ohio	x					x					
Oklahoma		x					x				
Oregon	x					x					
Pennsylvania				x					x		
Rhode Island				x					x		
South Carolina				x					x		
South Dakota				x					x		
Tennessee	x					x					
Texas				x					x		
Utah	x					x					
Vermont				x					x		

(continued)

Table 2 State Reporting Practice of COVID-19 Case and Death Data for NHPI Populations *(continued)*

State	COVID-19 cases					COVID-19 deaths					
	Reporting disaggregated NHPI data	Uses obsolete panracial "Asian Pacific Islander" category	Specifies NHPI data under "other" race category	Does not specify NHPI reporting practice	Does not report any race/ ethnicity data	Reporting disaggregated NHPI data	Uses obsolete panracial "Asian Pacific Islander" category	Specifies NHPI data under "other" race category	Does not specify NHPI reporting practice	Does not report any race/ ethnicity data	Does not report disaggregated NHPI death data
Virginia		x					x				
Washington	x					x					
West Virginia				x					x		
Wisconsin		x					x				
Wyoming	x					x					
Total	21	8	5	15	1	18	8	5	14	1	4
Percent	42	16	10	30	2	36	16	10	28	2	8

Table 3 Number and Percentage of California Counties with Underrepresented Racial/Ethnic Groups in the 4th Quartile of the California Healthy Places Index; N = 43 Counties

	Number of counties where that group is underrepresented in the 4th HPI quartile	% of counties where that group is underrepresented in the 4th HPI quartile
Hispanic or Latino	3	7%
Not Hispanic white alone	38	88%
Not Hispanic Black alone	15	35%
Not Hispanic AIAN alone	16	37%
Not Hispanic Asian alone	34	79%
Not Hispanic NHPI alone	21	49%

Note: AIAN = American Indian or Alaska Native.

underrepresenting Asian populations compared to the county's total population's percentage that reside within bottom-quartile census tracts. NHPIs were the second most affected, with 22 (49%) of 43 counties underrepresenting NHPI populations in bottom-quartile census tracts. American Indian/Alaska Native populations are underrepresented in 16 (37%) of 43 counties in the bottom-quartile census tracts. Latino/Hispanic populations were generally overrepresented in the majority of 4th-quartile tracts ranked by the HPI. Table 4 lists the California counties that underrepresent communities of color in the 4th quartile of the HPI, out of the 29 counties with populations greater than 150,000 people. The counties that underrepresent Asian, NHPI, American Indian/Alaska Native, and Black populations are listed separately for each racial group.

Discussion

Members of the NHPI community have long advocated for greater representation in data as an issue of data equity (Chang, Penaia, and Thomas 2020; Office of Hawaiian Affairs 1982; OMB 1997; Panapasa, Crabbe, and Kaholokula 2011). Disaggregated NHPI data are instrumental in supporting program implementation and policy advocacy to address long-standing social and health inequities. On the other hand, omissions of NHPI data through data-collection gaps or inappropriate aggregation of data in reporting are a form of structural racism and an extension of settler colonialism that stymies the passage and implementation of more inclusive public

Table 4 List of California Counties with Underrepresented Racial/Ethnic Communities of Color in the 4th Quartile of the California Healthy Places Index among 29 Counties with Populations Greater Than 150,000

Asian (25 counties)	NHPI (17 counties)	AIAN (12 counties)	Black (10 counties)
Los Angeles	Los Angeles	Los Angeles	Orange
San Diego	San Diego	San Bernardino	Santa Clara
Orange	Riverside	Fresno	Stanislaus
Riverside	Alameda	Kern	Tulare
San Bernardino	Contra Costa	Ventura	Santa Barbara
Santa Clara	Kern	San Joaquin	Monterey
Alameda	Ventura	Tulare	Placer
Contra Costa	San Joaquin	Santa Barbara	Santa Cruz
Fresno	Stanislaus	Placer	Imperial
Kern	Santa Barbara	San Luis Obispo	Kings
Ventura	Solano	Santa Cruz	
San Joaquin	Monterey	Madera	
Stanislaus	Placer		
Tulare	San Luis Obispo		
Santa Barbara	Santa Cruz		
Solano	Butte		
Monterey	Shasta		
Placer			
San Luis Obispo			
Santa Cruz			
Merced			
Yolo			
Imperial			
Madera			
Kings			

Note: AIAN = American Indian or Alaska Native.

policies (Morey et al. 2020; Tuck and Yang 2012). This article represents a review of publicly available data at the national, state, and local levels that could support public health and public policy efforts intended to benefit NHPI populations through data disaggregation in accordance with the revised OMB 15 standards. By reviewing these data, we aimed to evaluate the current state of data equity for NHPIs.

Our analysis of US federal data compliance with the revised OMB 15 standard for reporting NHPIs separately from Asian Americans found that there has indeed been progress since these same datasets were reviewed 10 years ago by Panapasa, Crabbe, and Kaholokula (2011). Our findings that some federal datasets that were not previously reporting disaggregated NHPI data are now in compliance with the revised OMB 15 standards indicate the success of many years of advocacy efforts by NHPI community members. Nevertheless, there is still work to be done. This is especially true of health data from the Department of Health and Human Services. Seven out of 13 federal health data sources are not reporting NHPI data separately from other racial/ethnic groups. One health data source, the Web-based Injury Statistics Query and Reporting System (WISQARS), is not collecting NHPI data in accordance with the revised OMB 15 standards. The remaining gaps in reporting are likely the result of insufficient sample sizes among the datasets that are collecting disaggregated NHPI data but not reporting the data. Many population-based samples, especially for health surveys, are limited in their reporting of NHPI data because they do not collect large enough samples of NHPIs to report the data publicly (Panapasa, Crabbe, and Kaholokula 2011).

Small sample sizes among NHPIs are a long-standing problem, as statistical estimates resulting from these small samples are often unstable. Confidentiality is a potential problem that limits the release of data for a small number of people who may be identifiable. At times, sufficiently large sample sizes can be obtained for NHPIs by pooling data across multiple years of data collection (Subica et al. 2017). However, such efforts often require accessing the restricted data files for these federal datasets. Accessing restricted data is not easy and is at times impossible because of confidentiality concerns. There are financial, time, geographic, and skill set barriers that prevent most researchers from enduring the arduous process of accessing restricted federal data. Therefore, researchers and data analysts studying relatively small and underresourced populations, such as NHPIs, must pay greater penalties to access the data they need, which may also underrepresent the needs of the population. There have been efforts to mitigate this problem. For example, the NHPI NHIS in 2014 collected a separate nationally representative NHPI sample to estimate the prevalence of disease in this population for the first time (National Center for Health Statistics 2014). We recognize that there are greater financial costs of oversampling smaller populations. Nevertheless, these costs are outweighed by the health, societal, and financial costs associated with overlooking inequities for minoritized populations, which become compounded over time. More efforts are needed to make sure

NHPIs are included in nationally representative surveys and that collected data are made available for the public to access to inform policy decisions.

Timely and transparent data are extremely important to inform public health efforts, especially during a global pandemic. As the COVID-19 pandemic has shown, the numbers are constantly changing, as are the corresponding scientific and policy recommendations. From the early days of the pandemic, states and counties were reporting extremely high rates of COVID-19 cases and deaths among NHPI populations (Chang, Penaia, and Thomas 2020; Morey et al. 2020). The formation of the NHPI Data Policy Lab allowed for these data to be consolidated and disseminated, supporting local, state, and national efforts to garner resources to address the disproportionate effects of COVID-19 on NHPI populations (Samoa et al. 2020). As the NHPI Data Policy Lab Dashboard shows, NHPI populations continue to be greatly impacted by the pandemic, with the highest rates of COVID-19 cases and deaths among all racial/ethnic groups in the majority of states that report NHPI data (UCLA Center on Health Policy Research 2021). Although NHPI populations are found in all 50 states, most states are not disaggregating NHPI case and death data. It is unclear how NHPI data are being specified in some states. Eight states are reporting NHPI data with Asian data in a panracial "Asian Pacific Islander" category, while five states are consolidating NHPI data in the "other race" category.

Using the panracial "Asian Pacific Islander" category violates the revised OMB 15 standards and inflicts harm on NHPI communities (OMB 1997; Panapasa, Crabbe, and Kaholokula 2011). Although we recognize that NHPI and Asian panracial coalitions continue to collaborate to achieve common goals, when it comes to directing public resources to address social and health problems, more data disaggregation for NHPI and Asian subpopulations is crucial. In states where the majority of Asian Americans are experiencing lower COVID-19 case and death rates and also make up a larger proportion of the population than NHPIs, the plight of NHPIs is obscured, hiding disparities (Chang, Penaia, and Thomas 2020; Ponce, Shimkhada, and Tulua 2021). In North Carolina, data were showing that NHPIs were experiencing the highest COVID-19 death rates in the state. However, for reasons unknown, the state began aggregating NHPIs with Asian Americans, thus hiding the disparity within the racial group currently experiencing the lowest death rates in the state (UCLA Center for Health Policy Research 2021). Therefore, aggregating NHPIs with Asian Americans commits harm against NHPI communities, limiting their ability to advocate for resources to combat the pandemic. In a situation as dire as the COVID-19 pandemic, disaggregated NHPI data are desperately needed to mobilize efforts to save lives. This is why even though statisticians and epidemiologists have cited problems with small numbers, including potential anonymity issues, NHPI advocates have been calling for the release of NHPI COVID-19 case and death data as a separate race category, regardless of the size of the numbers (Morey et al. 2020; Samoa et al. 2020). The handling of NHPI COVID-19 data influences life-and-death decisions about whether NHPI communities are included in plans for equitable COVID-19 response.

The exclusion of NHPIs in equity plans to combat the COVID-19 pandemic becomes clear at the local level. In the state of California, the HPI is being used to inform the distribution of COVID-19 resources—including vaccines—to the neighborhoods considered most disadvantaged (Lin II, Money, and Shalby 2021). However, our analysis shows that the HPI underrepresents NHPI populations, even while NHPI populations are experiencing the highest COVID-19 case rate (10,572 per 100,000) and death rate (204 per 100,000) in California compared to all other race and ethnic groups. While the HPI by design does not include neighborhood data on race/ethnicity because of Proposition 209, its purpose is to allocate resources to the areas most affected by the pandemic. In the case of NHPI populations who are suffering in the pandemic, the HPI underrepresents them. This may be due in part to NHPI and other smaller populations such as American Indians/Alaska Natives being more spread out and less concentrated than larger minoritized populations experiencing residential segregation. Furthermore, place-based measures may systematically bias against socioeconomic dimensions of household composition. The HPI measures socioeconomic status using median household income, which is artificially inflated for NHPI households, which tend to be large, multigenerational, and multifamily (Delaney et al. 2018). This unintended bias against NHPI communities embedded in neighborhood socioeconomic measures is a form of structural racism. In the absence of allowing race data in California to be considered as part of a plan for equitable distribution of resources because of Proposition 209, other metrics might be more relevant to capture neighborhood risk for groups such as NHPIs in equity metrics such as the HPI. For example, per capita income can be used instead of median household income, which will address the problem of underestimating the socioeconomic needs of families living in large multifamily homes with several income earners.

The underestimation of NHPI needs by only focusing on the most disadvantaged neighborhoods identified by area-level metrics like the HPI demonstrates a form of structural racism that often persists unnoticed (California Pan-Ethnic Health Network 2021). Increasingly, health organizations in the government, nonprofit, and for-profit realms are relying on similar metrics and thresholds to make decisions about how to target resources. The availability of big data allows for these types of metrics to be created and used widely, with concrete consequences. Recent research has shown decisions that are "race neutral" on the surface can end up unjustly disadvantaging communities of color and propagating societal biases (Obermeyer et al. 2019; Zou and Schiebinger 2018). Although California Proposition 209 was originally marketed as a civil rights initiative to make public policy decisions in a "color blind" way, evidence from this study and others has shown that when public and private institutions ignore race/ethnicity completely, conscious and unconscious biases against communities of color proliferate (Kidder 2013). Most of the time, the average consumer is unaware of how these metrics work or how they were developed, even though they may have serious implications for health and social equity. Therefore, we shed light on the potential weaknesses of the large-scale use of some metrics to determine the allocation of resources that may disadvantage the communities of color that need the most resources to combat racial injustices, including NHPIs. We recognize that there is great potential with the increasing use of big data to make program and policy decisions using health equity metrics. At the same time, we caution that these metrics must be applied with transparency and with deliberate attention paid to the problems of racial inequity that can result from their use (Green 2020).

Recommendations

Having demonstrated the importance of data equity as fundamental to achieving social and health justice for NHPIs, we provide the following recommendations. First, at the national, state, and local levels data must be collected and reported in accordance with the revised OMB 15 guidelines set in 1997 wherever this is not already occurring. All systems currently collecting race data should be collecting data for NHPIs separately from Asian Americans and from other race categories. This is the same call to action that has been ongoing for decades (Chang, Penaia, and Thomas 2020; Office of Hawaiian Affairs 1982; Panapasa, Crabbe, and Kaholokula

2011). Every effort should be made to report disaggregated NHPI data and to make these data easily and publicly accessible, in accordance with the revised OMB 15 standards. As a majority of NHPIs are multiracial but also strongly identify being NHPI, we recommend that statisticians consider including multiracial NHPIs in a separate "multiracial NHPI" category or in the larger NHPI category. This should be done with transparency, noting how data for multiracial people are being treated. Although epidemiologists and statisticians often hesitate to report the small numbers for NHPIs because of unstable rates or not reaching a certain statistical threshold, we contend that the data should be reported anyway, with caveats outlining the limitations of the data. As in the case of the COVID-19 pandemic, these numbers were essential in the early days of the crisis to mobilize grassroots community responses to the spread of the virus, even when the initial numbers were low (Samoa et al. 2020). Making data more transparent allows communities to make informed decisions and to understand how their data are being treated. The agencies collecting population data should realize the power that they wield when making decisions about which data to make publicly available. NHPIs and other relatively smaller populations have a higher transaction cost to access their own community's data. Therefore, agencies should make efforts to lower these costs for communities who, like NHPIs, are underrepresented so that community researchers have equitable and ethical access to data.

Second, recognizing that the sample sizes of NHPIs collected at the federal level are often not large enough to be reportable or to inform decisions, we recommend a second round of NHPI NHIS data collection. The 2014 NHPI NHIS has been extensively used to report on NHPI disparities (Narcisse et al. 2020). A subsequent iteration of the NHPI NHIS will bolster the sample size and provide more accurate surveillance of NHPI health nationally.

Third, when possible, NHPI data should be further disaggregated into subpopulations given the diverse languages, cultural practices, and histories of each of the Pacific Island groups that have been impacted by settler colonialism, militarization, and migration in ways distinct from one another. For example, Native Hawaiians have experienced the historical trauma of having lands and culture stripped away by the US government (Dougherty 1992; Kaholokula et al. 2020; Ong 2009). Pacific Islanders from Federated States of Micronesia, Republic of Marshall Islands, and Republic of Palau who are under the Compacts of Free Association

(COFA) were subjected to severe health consequences and loss of land as a result of the US government's nuclear testing on the islands from 1946 to 1958. Although COFA migrants are allowed to live and work in the United States,[11] they were denied access to Medicaid under the 1996 Personal Responsibility and Work Opportunity Reconciliation Act until Congress restored Medicaid access in December 2020 (Asian and Pacific Islander American Health Forum 2020; McElfish, Hallgren, and Yamada 2015). Chamorros, the Indigenous people of Guam, have survived centuries of settler colonialism, first by Spain and then by the United States as an unincorporated territory, and their territory is used as a military outpost.[12] Although people born and living on Guam are considered US citizens, they are denied constitutional protections such as the right to vote in presidential elections. American Sāmoa has had a similar history of militarization and settler colonialism as an unincorporated US territory. American Sāmoans are considered US nationals and must go through the naturalization process to earn the rights of US citizenship, such as applying for certain jobs or voting in presidential elections (Asian Americans Advancing Justice 2014).[13] Although we cannot illuminate each unique story of the many Pacific Islands here, we provide these few examples to demonstrate how various historical contexts and political forces differentially shape the well-being and social standing of NHPI subpopulations in the United States. Therefore, fine-grained data are needed to highlight the diversity within the NHPI aggregate grouping.

Fourth, stronger partnerships are needed between government, academic, and community-based organizations to increase NHPI sample

11. This is another example of settler colonialism operating. The land and waters were seen as a valuable military outpost to be used for nuclear testing to advance US power, while the people were treated as expendable. COFA serves to continue this legacy of settler colonialism, displacing Pacific Islanders from their native lands in exchange for the United States having continued access to the islands for military purposes, simultaneously exploiting COFA migrants' bodies and labor in the United States.

12. Another example of militarization, Guam was long under rule by the US Navy, while Chamorros were often treated as expendable by the US government. For example, during World War II, Guam was bombed and seized by Japan only hours after the bombing of Pearl Harbor, leading to the suffering and death of many Chamorros (see *Cultures of Commemoration: The Politics of War, Memory and History in the Mariana Islands* by Keith L. Camacho).

13. American Sāmoa is the only unincorporated US territory where people born there are not automatically considered US citizens. A recent (June 15, 2021) federal appeals court ruled that US citizenship should not be forced on American Sāmoans. This is in response to a lower court ruling siding with three people from American Sāmoa who sued to be recognized as US citizens. Some government leaders and community members in American Sāmoa have fought against automatic citizenship, which could disrupt traditions of communal land ownership. Still others argue that the naturalization path is too costly for American Sāmoans.

sizes and to make data more useful. Institutions should listen to and learn from NHPI voices to understand the types of data outputs that will be most appropriate and to make data-collection efforts more effective. Egalitarian relationships, open communication, and sensitive outreach to NHPI community organizations will allow for the improvement of data collection and quality. Furthermore, institutions of higher education and national funders should invest in building capacity among NHPI community organizations to support the next generation of researchers and data scientists who understand the specific needs of NHPI populations. Building stronger infrastructure within the NHPI community will enable grassroots efforts to use data to inform policy and programmatic solutions. Such commitments will help to mitigate the systemic underinvestment in communities of color such as NHPIs.

Fifth, we recognize that in the era of big data and machine learning, summary metrics can be inherently biased against people of color, especially populations such as NHPIs who are underrepresented in data systems to begin with. Therefore, we recommend that future metrics must be created with a careful and deliberate focus on equity (Green 2020). The consideration of equity should apply broadly to communities of color, including NHPI populations. Metrics used to determine distribution of resources must be made transparent to allow the public to evaluate whether these metrics are truly effective and equitable. As such metrics are being created and applied increasingly widely, we recommend the purposeful evaluation of the effects of using these metrics for public policy decisions on racial equity. People creating and applying these metrics must be educated on issues of racial equity. These steps will help to ensure that policy decisions made based on these metrics do not perpetuate and exacerbate racial biases that exist in society.

Conclusion

We recognize the great progress that has been made in the collection and reporting of data for NHPI populations in the United States, largely because of the grassroots efforts and advocacy that have been ongoing from NHPI community members for decades. However, our work is far from complete. We continue to advocate for the appropriate disaggregation of NHPI data to achieve equity. By achieving data equity, our hope is that future generations will be able to achieve health and social equity for all communities of color.

■ ■ ■

Brittany N. Morey is an assistant professor with the Department of Health, Society, and Behavior at the University of California, Irvine. She also is a faculty affiliate with the NHPI Data Policy Lab at the UCLA Center for Health Policy Research. Her research focuses on how structural inequity shapes racial and ethnic health inequities, the overall goal of which is to understand how society creates health inequities along the lines of race/ethnicity, nativity, and immigration status to inform better policies and programs that address and undo these patterns.
brittany.morey@uci.edu

Richard Calvin Chang is the data analytics director and a cofounding member of the NHPI Data Policy Lab at the UCLA Center for Health Policy Research. His work focuses on raising awareness of COVID-19's disproportionate impact on NHPIs and ensuring the community is accurately represented with policy makers and stakeholders. He previously worked as an attorney and policy director for NHPI nonprofits and served as president of the Pacific Islander Health Partnership. He is a coauthor of the first demographic profile of NHPIs and "Policy Platform Blueprint for Native Hawaiians and Pacific Islanders in the United States."

Karla Blessing Thomas is the policy director and a cofounding member of the NHPI Data Policy Lab at the UCLA Center for Health Policy Research. She is a community activist passionate about advancing health equity for Pacific Islanders, and she currently leads community-based COVID-19 response efforts in California's Inland Empire.

'Alisi Tulua is the project director of the NHPI Data Policy Lab at the UCLA Center for Health Policy Research. She brings her 15-plus years of nonprofit experience serving NHPI communities to her current role, which focuses on building data capacity for promoting health equity for NHPIs.

Corina Penaia is the community engagement and research director and a cofounding member of the NHPI Data Policy Lab at the UCLA Center for Health Policy Research. She works closely with policy makers and community stakeholders to address prevalent health issues that impact Pacific Islander and Asian families. Her experience includes implementing public health programs in underserved communities, where she has developed a passion for and extensive expertise in producing culturally relevant and sensitive programming centered on food insecurity, chronic diseases, and related policy and advocacy as well as implementing nutrition education and obesity prevention programs.

Vananh D. Tran is a third-year medical student at the David Geffen School of Medicine at UCLA and is part of the Program in Medical Education—Leadership and Advocacy (PRIME-LA). Her academic interests lie in the intersection of medicine, inequity, policy, and health.

Nicholas Pierson is a former high school teacher and a current data scientist with the NHPI Data Policy Lab at the UCLA Center for Health Policy Research.

John C. Greer is a data scientist with the NHPI Data Policy Lab at the UCLA Center for Health Policy Research. His work focuses on building data systems that highlight the impact of COVID-19 on NHPIs.

Malani Bydalek is a graduate of UC Irvine whose primary interests lie in environmental justice and conservation.

Ninez Ponce is professor with the UCLA Fielding School of Public Health and a director at the UCLA Center for Health Policy Research. She leads the California Health Interview Survey, the nation's largest state health survey that is recognized as a national model for race/ethnicity data collection. She has served on committees for the National Center for Health Statistics and the National Academy of Medicine, where her expertise has focused on the measurement and use of race/ethnicity to monitor health equity. In 2019 she received AcademyHealth's HSR Impact Award for her contributions to population health measurement to inform public policies.

Acknowledgments

This work was supported by grants from the Robert Wood Johnson Foundation (grant #79504, "A Model for Data-Driven Policy Making in the NHPI Community") and the National Institute on Minority Health and Health Disparities (NIH R01 MD012292). We acknowledge and thank Sela V. Panapasa, Kamana'opono M. Crabbe, and Joseph Keawe'aimoku Kaholokula for their original examination of federal data compliance with the 1997 revised OMB 15 standards for collecting and reporting NHPI data.

References

Asian Americans Advancing Justice. 2014. "A Community of Contrasts: Native Hawaiians and Pacific Islanders in the United States." www.advancingjustice-aajc.org/sites/default/files/2016-09/2014_Community%20of%20Contrasts.pdf (accessed October 19, 2021).

Asian and Pacific Islander American Health Forum. 2020. "Medicaid Restoration for Compact of Free Association Communities." www.apiahf.org/focus/health-care-access/cofa/ (accessed June 19, 2021).

Bailey, Zinzi D., Nancy Krieger, Madina Agénor, Jasmine Graves, Natalia Linos, and Mary T. Bassett. 2017. "Structural Racism and Health Inequities in the USA: Evidence and Interventions." *Lancet* 389, no. 10077: 1453–63. doi.org/10.1016/S0140-6736(17)30569-X.

California Pan-Ethnic Health Network. 2021. "Nothing About Us Without Us: Can Area-Based Social Indices Effectively Advance Health Equity?" October 26. cpehn.org/publications/nothing-about-us-without-us/

Chang, Richard Calvin, Corina Penaia, and Karla Thomas. 2020. "Count Native Hawaiian and Pacific Islanders in COVID-19 Data—It's an OMB Mandate." *Health Affairs Blog*, August 27. www.healthaffairs.org/do/10.1377/hblog20200825.671245/full/.

"The COVID Tracking Project." 2021. *Atlantic*. covidtracking.com/ (accessed October 19, 2021).

Delaney, Tracy, Will Dominie, Helen Dowling, Neil Maizlish, Derek Chapman, Latoya Hill, Christine Orndahl, et al. 2018. "The California Healthy Places Index." Public Health Alliance of Southern California. healthyplacesindex.org (accessed October 19, 2021).

Diez Roux, Ana V., and Christina Mair. 2010. "Neighborhoods and Health." *Annals of the New York Academy of Sciences* 1186, no. 1: 125–45.

Dougherty, Michael. 1992. *To Steal a Kingdom: Probing Hawaiian History*. Waimanalo, HI: Island Style Press.

Gee, Gilbert C., and Chandra L. Ford. 2011. "Structural Racism and Health Inequities." *Du Bois Review: Social Science Research on Race* 8, no. 1: 115–32.

Green, Ben. 2020. "Data Science as Political Action: Grounding Data Science in a Politics of Justice." *SSRN*, August 29. dx.doi.org/10.2139/ssrn.3658431.

Hawai'i Department of Health. 2021. "Hawai'i COVID-19 Summary Metrics." Hawai'i COVID-19 Data. health.hawaii.gov/coronavirusdisease2019/what-you-should-know/current-situation-in-hawaii/ (accessed October 19, 2021).

Hixson, Lindsay, Bradford B. Hepler, and Myoung Ouk Kim. 2012. "The Native Hawaiian and Other Pacific Islander Population: 2010." US Census Bureau, Report #C2010BR-12, May. www.census.gov/library/publications/2012/dec/c2010br-12.html#:~:text=According%20to%20the%202010%20Census,one%20or%20more%20other%20races.

Hosaka, Kalei R. J., Max P. Castanera, and Seiji Yamada. 2021. "Structural Racism and Micronesians in Hawaii: The COVID-19 Syndemic." *Asia Pacific Journal of Public Health*, May 3. doi.org/10.1177/10105395211012188.

Kaholokula, Joseph Keawe'aimoku, Robin E. S. Miyamoto, Andrea Hepuapo'okela Hermosura, and Megan Inada. 2020. "Prejudice, Stigma, and Oppression on the Behavioral Health of Native Hawaiians and Pacific Islanders." In *Prejudice, Stigma, Privilege, and Oppression: A Behavioral Health Handbook*, edited by Lorraine T. Benuto, Melanie P. Duckworth, Akihiko Matsuda, and William O'Donohue, 107–34. New York: Springer.

Kana'iaupuni, Shawn Malia. 2011. "Lots of Aloha, Little Data: Data and Research on Native Hawaiian and Pacific Islanders." *AAPI Nexus: Policy, Practice, and Community* 9, nos. 1–2: 207–11.

Kidder, William C. 2013. "Misshaping the River: Proposition 209 and Lessons for the Fisher Case." *Journal of College and University Law* 39, no. 1: 53–127.

Lin, Rong-Gong II, Luke Money, and Colleen Shalby. 2021. "California Is Reserving 40% of COVID-19 Vaccine for the Neediest. Who Will Get It?" *Los Angeles Times*, March 4. www.latimes.com/california/story/2021-03-04/california-shifts-covid-vaccine-rollout-for-neediest-groups.

Maizlish, Neil, Tracy Delaney, Helen Dowling, Derek A. Chapman, Roy Sabo, Steven Woolf, Christine Orndahl, Latoya Hill, and Lauren Snellings. 2019. "California Healthy Places Index: Frames Matter." *Public Health Reports* 134, no. 4: 354–62. doi.org/10.1177/0033354919849882.

McElfish, Pearl Anna, Emily Hallgren, and Seiji Yamada. 2015. "Effect of US Health Policies on Health Care Access for Marshallese Migrants." *American Journal of Public Health* 105, no. 4: 637–43. doi.org/10.2105/AJPH.2014.302452.

Morey, Brittany N. 2014. "Environmental Justice for Native Hawaiians and Pacific Islanders in Los Angeles County." *Environmental Justice* 7, no. 1: 9–17.

Morey, Brittany N., ʻAlisi Tulua, Sora Park Tanjasiri, Andrew M. Subica, Joseph Keaweʻaimoku Kaholokula, Corina Penaia, Karla Thomas, et al. 2020. "Structural Racism and Its Effects on Native Hawaiians and Pacific Islanders in the United States: Issues of Health Equity, Census Undercounting, and Voter Disenfranchisement." *AAPI Nexus: Policy, Practice, and Community*, October 24. www.aapinexus.org/2020/11/24/structural-racism-and-its-effects-on-native-hawaiians-and-pacific-islanders.

Narcisse, Marie-R., Page Dobbs, Christopher R. Long, Rachel S. Purvis, Kim S. Kimminau, and Pearl A. McElfish. 2020. "Electronic Cigarette Use and Psychological Distress in the Native Hawaiian and Pacific Islander Adults Compared with Other Racial/Ethnic Groups: Data from the National Health Interview Survey, 2014." *Journal of Community Psychology* 48, no. 2: 225–36. doi.org/10.1002/jcop.22248.

National Center for Health Statistics. 2014. "Native Hawaiian and Pacific Islander (NHPI) National Health Interview Survey." Centers for Disease Control and Prevention. www.cdc.gov/nchs/nhis/nhpi.html (accessed October 10, 2021).

Obermeyer, Ziad, Brian Powers, Christine Vogeli, and Sendhil Mullainathan. 2019. "Dissecting Racial Bias in an Algorithm Used to Manage the Health of Populations." *Science* 366, no. 6464: 447–53. doi.org/10.1126/science.aax2342.

Office of Hawaiian Affairs. 1982. "Office of Hawaiian Affair's Goals, Objectives, and Policies." In *OHA Master Plan*, n.p. Honolulu: Office of Hawaiian Affairs.

Okamoto, Dina, and G. Christina Mora. 2014. "Panethnicity." *Annual Review of Sociology* 40, no. 1: 219–39.

OMB (Office of Management and Budget). 1997. "Revisions to the Standards for the Classification of Federal Data on Race and Ethnicity." *Federal Register*, October 30. www.federalregister.gov/documents/1997/10/30/97-28653/revisions-to-the-standards-for-the-classification-of-federal-data-on-race-and-ethnicity.

Ong, Paul. 2009. "Trouble in Paradise: The Economic Marginalization of Native Hawaiians." In *Wealth Accumulation and Communities of Color in the United States: Current Issues*, edited by Jessica Gordon Nembhard and Ngina Chiteji, 155–72. Ann Arbor: University of Michigan Press.

Panapasa, Sela V., Kamanaʻopono M. Crabbe, and Joseph Keaweʻaimoku Kaholokula. 2011. "Efficacy of Federal Data: Revised Office of Management and Budget Standard for Native Hawaiian and Other Pacific Islanders Examined." *AAPI Nexus* 9, nos. 1–2: 212–20.

Pastor, Manuel, and Rachel Morello-Frosch. 2014. "Integrating Public Health and Community Development to Tackle Neighborhood Distress and Promote Well-Being." *Health Affairs* 33, no. 11: 1890–96. doi.org/10.1377/hlthaff.2014.0640.

Ponce, Ninez A., Riti Shimkhada, and ʻAlisi Tulua. 2021. "Disaggregating California's COVID-19 Data for Native Hawaiians and Pacific Islanders and Asians." UCLA Center for Health Policy Research, May 26. healthpolicy.ucla.edu/publications/search/pages/detail.aspx?PubID=2135.

Public Health Alliance of Southern California. 2021. "Data and Reports." healthyplacesindex.org/data-reports/ (accessed October 19, 2021).

Reskin, Barbara. 2012. "The Race Discrimination System." *Annual Review of Sociology* 38, no. 1: 17–35. doi.org/10.1146/annurev-soc-071811-145508.

Samoa, Raynald, Joseph Keaweʻaimoku Kaholokula, Corina Penaia, Ridvan Tupai-Firestone, Elena Faʻamoe-Timoteo, Melisa Leaelan, and Nia Aitaoto. 2020. "COVID-19 and the State of Health of Pacific Islanders in the United States." *AAPI Nexus: Policy, Practice, and Community*, September 24. www.aapinexus.org/2020/09/24/article-covid-19-and-the-state-of-health-of-pacific-islanders-in-the-united-states/.

Subica, Andrew M., Neha Agarwal, J. Greer Sullivan, and Bruce G. Link. 2017. "Obesity and Associated Health Disparities among Understudied Multiracial, Pacific Islander, and American Indian Adults." *Obesity* 25, no. 12: 2128–36. doi.org/10.1002/oby.21954.

Taualii, Maile, Joey Quenga, Raynald Samoa, Salim Samanani, and Doug Dover. 2011. "Liberating Data: Accessing Native Hawaiian and Other Pacific Islander Data from National Data Sets." *AAPI Nexus* 9, nos. 1–2: 249–55.

Tuck, Eve, and K. Wayne Yang. 2012. "Decolonization Is Not a Metaphor." *Decolonization: Indigeneity, Education, and Society* 1, no. 1: 1–40.

UCLA Center for Health Policy Research. 2021. "NHPI COVID-19 Data Policy Lab Dashboard." UCLA Fielding School of Public Health. healthpolicy.ucla.edu/health-profiles/Pages/NHPI-COVID-19-Dashboard.aspx (accessed October19, 2021).

US Census Bureau. 2020. "American Community Survey 2015–2019 5-Year Data Release." December 10. www.census.gov/newsroom/press-kits/2020/acs-5-year.html.

Zou, James, and Londa Schiebinger. 2018. "AI Can Be Sexist and Racist—It's Time to Make It Fair." *Nature*, July 18. www.nature.com/articles/d41586-018-05707-8.

The Political Realignment of Health: How Partisan Power Shaped Infant Health in the United States, 1915–2017

Javier M. Rodríguez
Byengseon Bae
Claremont Graduate University

Arline T. Geronimus
John Bound
University of Michigan

Abstract The US two-party system was transformed in the 1960s when the Democratic Party abandoned its Jim Crow protectionism to incorporate the policy agenda fostered by the civil rights movement, and the Republican Party redirected its platform toward socioeconomic and racial conservatism. The authors argue that the policy agendas promoted by the two parties through presidents and state legislatures codify a racially patterned access to resources and power detrimental to the health of all. To test the hypothesis that fluctuations in overall and race-specific infant mortality rates (IMRs) shift between the parties in power before and after the political realignment (PR), the authors apply panel data analysis methods to state-level data from the National Center for Health Statistics for the period 1915 through 2017. Net of trend, overall, and race-specific IMRs were not statistically different between presidential parties before the PR. This pattern, however, changed after the PR, with Republican administrations consistently underperforming Democratic ones. Net of trend, non-Southern state legislatures controlled by Republicans underperform Democratic ones in overall and racial IMRs in both periods.

Keywords institutional racism, political parties, infant mortality, health disparities, policy

Although key public health indicators have dramatically improved over the past century, racial disparities in health have remained entrenched. In the early 1900s, Black infants and mothers died at almost twice the rate of their white counterparts; by the early 2000s, although overall rates had declined in both groups over the century, the Black excess deaths increased to about 2.5 times the rate of whites for infants, and 3.5 times for mothers. Research

Journal of Health Politics, Policy and Law, Vol. 47, No. 2, April 2022
DOI 10.1215/03616878-9517191

on maternal and infant health inequity over the 20th century has disproportionately focused on maternal demographic, behavioral, and health care access risks during pregnancy. Experiences of interpersonal racism, perceived unfair treatment, and race-related stress have been added to the range of personal experiences that can negatively affect pregnancy outcomes (Ertel et al. 2012; Williams 2002). Yet, less attention has been paid to the role of structural racism (Almond, Chay, and Greenstone 2006; Bhatia, Krieger, and Subramanian 2019; Geronimus 1992, 2000) and the political processes through which it is maintained in shaping population health inequity (Cottrell et al. 2019; Rodriguez 2019). Accordingly, this study contributes to this agenda by arguing that structural racism is fundamentally political. This is because structural racism represents the web of interconnected, mutually reinforcing institutional systems that differentially produce and distribute social and health outcomes by race, and such systems are bounded by policy, law, and the practices that result from official norms, rules, and regulations—all of which are exclusive to government activity.

Party Control of the Presidency and State Legislatures

Rodriguez, Bound, and Geronimus (2014a, 2014b) documented a robust association, net of secular trend, between the party of the US president and infant mortality rates (IMRs) since 1965, whereby infants fared better under Democratic presidencies than Republican ones. Similarly, Rodriguez and colleagues (2021) analyzed state-level data from 1969 through 2014 to report a powerful net-of-trend association between infant mortality indicators and the party controlling lower and upper chambers in state legislatures as well as the overall state legislature. Focusing at the state level, here too infants fared better under Democratic-controlled state legislatures than Republican ones, with effects even larger than those reported for presidents. While precise mechanisms remain to be explicated, these findings suggest that federal and state governments in the United States are powerful institutions shaping the social determinants of health—for example, education, income, housing, the built environment, social context, and access to and quality of health care services—and suggest that larger mutable political processes constitute components of the underlying mechanism generating US population inequities in pregnancy outcomes.

Given that their identified trends were from time series beginning in the 1960s, Rodriguez and colleagues speculated that the policy polarization that emerged from the political realignment (PR) of the Democratic and

Republican parties after the civil rights movement, the centrality of race in the PR, the different size and nature of the social welfare safety net promoted by the parties, and their views toward a competitive health care system might be explanatory. If that interpretation is correct, we would not expect to see the same dramatic differences in net-of-trend IMRs by party of the president before the realignment.

Parties and Race before and after the PR

The US two-party system was transformed at the national level in the 1960s, when the Democratic Party abandoned its Jim Crow protectionism to incorporate the policy agenda fostered by the civil rights movement, and the Republican Party redirected its policy platform from one that was less conservative on civil rights and racial issues toward a fierce and racially coded economic and social conservatism. This dramatic shift in national partisan policy was actually a realignment across numerous political elements (Clubb, Flanigan, and Zingale 1980). It was accompanied by deep changes in partisan lobbying, coalitional, institutional, and constituent bases—the ones capable of disrupting the political environment that generates durable electoral groupings and partisan-polarizing events (Beck 1974; Burnham 1970, 1975; Key 1955). As the PR advanced, race became the most important issue around which the parties reorganized and bonded together critical aspects of national government activity (Bartels and Cramer 2019; Carmines and Stimson 1989; Osborne, Sears, and Valentino 2011; Tesler 2016; Valentino and Sears 2005).

In the United States, political eras have rested on embedded ideologies of race, where the policy-making process, the policy agenda that results from it, and its execution shield the racial hierarchy that preserves the inequitable access to resources, power, and opportunity of a given era. Before the PR, racial discrimination in the form of a Jim Crow system existed in both legalized and nonlegalized forms since the post–Civil War era. Although de jure racism existed in both Southern and non-Southern states, Jim Crow laws were particularly rooted in the South, where a "one-party Democratic era" dominated this period (Heersink and Jenkins 2020). From the 1890s until 1944—when the US Supreme Court invalidated the "white only" Democratic primary in the 11 states of the old Confederacy—the Democratic Party operated in these states through authoritarian enclaves. During this period, the Democratic Party benefited from aggressive demobilization of the electorate and repression of their political opposition as well as from creating and policing racially segregated spheres of US society (Caughey 2018; Mickey 2008, 2015).

During this period both parties, nationally and at the state level, furthered the interests of white people. In addition, until the 1950s the Republican Party ("the party of Lincoln") at the national level was conservative on civil rights and racial issues. Still, the Democratic Party was the more conservative of the two parties on race. To achieve its political aims, the Democratic Party connected and exploited geographically grounded social and cultural unrests between the races in the South, from slavery to Jim Crow. The Democratic Party benefited from stringent electoral suppression via voter restrictions and the support of paramilitary groups terrorizing Black citizens and other minorities, while the Republican Party showed some biracial coalitions by the late 1890s. In some states, Republicans incorporated Black voters to elect white (and in some particular instances, Black) Republican officials since the Reconstruction era. Yet, the Republican Party almost disappeared from Southern politics. During the first half of the 20th century, Southern Republicans contributed a mere 3.2% of all US House representatives and not a single US senator (Heersink and Jenkins 2020). At the brink of political extinction in the South, the Republican Party saw the need for a drastic shift in its electoral appeal.

By the eve of the civil rights movement, the political dynamics between the two parties and their policy agendas were inherently racialized. As dissatisfaction with the civil rights movement grew among working-class whites in the 1950s, the Republican Party reworked national-level policies that preserved explicit racism from the previous eras into national policies that integrated an implicit—yet no less harmful—type of racism (Inwood 2015). By committing its national agenda to neoliberalism via policies for market deregulation, regressive tax cuts, small government, and shrinking the social safety net, the Republican Party broadened an economic argument that repackaged racism into US political economy (Inwood 2015).

Nationally, while the Republican Party incorporated a falsely colorblind macroeconomics agenda that, in effect, benefited white people over Black people, it simultaneously promulgated an ideology of meritocratic individualism—one that justified the continuing social hierarchy on the basis of personal effort rather than explaining it as an effect of structural racism (Sears and Henry 2003). At the same time, the national Democratic Party lost the support of poor and working-class whites, especially in the South, as it reengineered itself to support heavy public investment in health, infrastructure, and social welfare while opposing the budget cuts of new

Republican conservatives (Phillips 1970). The Vietnam War broke bipartisan consensus on foreign policy (Aldrich 1995), and Republicans unified efforts with conservative religious movements (Brennan 1995; Levendusky 2009). Pushing the boundaries of ideological preferences, both parties focused on cementing partisanship and party identification as a social identity (Green, Palmquist, and Schickler 2002). The national policy platforms of both parties were promoted as color-blind, even as they had racially disparate impacts (Bonilla-Silva 2006). Implicit racial conservatism was absorbed into ordinary policy forms of social and economic conservatism, therefore shaping "the conditions in which people are born, grow, live, work, and age"—that is, the social determinants of health (WHO 2008).

Beginning with John F. Kennedy and Lyndon B. Johnson during the civil rights movement era of the 1960s, it was Democratic presidents who settled the legal background for future government activity. Lyndon B. Johnson's unprecedented array of Great Society and War on Poverty programs framed the political course of the social determinants of health and their distribution by socioeconomic status and race. The size and scope of the Great Society and the War on Poverty programs to end social and racial injustice consisted of nearly 200 pieces of legislation addressing civil rights, poverty, education, health, immigration, the environment, housing, access to the financial system, and political participation, among others. A number of important executive orders were issued and acts signed into law in the early 1960s (e.g., Executive Order No. 10925 inaugurating affirmative action in 1961; the Equal Pay Act of 1963; and the Food Stamp Act, Elementary and Secondary Education Act, and Economic Opportunity Act of 1964).

But the turning point for health law happened in 1965 when at least 29 pieces of legislation passed, affecting population health from then onward. Of these, 15 laws explicitly reformed crucial determinants of health by expanding budgets for hospital equipment and facilities, improving planning and health care coordination, focusing on disease prevention and health education, and increasing access to and quality of health care services, among other effects (Forgotson 1967) (table 1A in the appendix describes these laws; for a detailed list of interventions historically affecting infant mortality in the United States since 1840 see Bhatia, Krieger, and Subramanian [2019]; see also KFF [2011]). Overall, the Great Society and War on Poverty programs shaped racial disparities in health. For example, the Civil Rights Act of 1964 and the Voting Rights Act of 1965 improved the sociopolitical status of Black individuals and other minorities. By officially forbidding job discrimination and the segregation of public accommodations, some social contexts became less stressful for minority communities.

Spillover effects from the War on Poverty improved racial minorities' health as they were more likely to be poor.

In many ways, Lyndon B. Johnson's policy expansions represented the continuation of the similarly dramatic array of policies and programs enacted by Franklin Delano Roosevelt to counteract the effects of the Great Depression. It was the New Deal—under the administration of a Democratic president—that made a political party the institutional base for ideological cohesion, cooperative federalism, and stronger top-down federal-state aid programs and activism, including coalitions with labor movement organizations and constituencies (e.g., the Congress of Industrial Organizations, Black voters in non-Southern states, and ethnic and immigrant communities like those from southern and eastern Europe) (Gerring 1998). In a period when state policy agendas operated more in tandem with local-level economic interests and coalitions than with national-level policy, the Democratic Party started to manifest a different behavior: its state policy platforms were getting "nationalized" and coordinated with platforms at the federal level, including far-reaching federal programs such as Social Security that carried provisions for maternal and child health (Johnson 1961).

In this sense, pre–World War II federalism and the two-party system looked more like loose coalitions of state- and local-level actors, where the two parties were interpreted as "semipublic associations" with organizational structures comprising highly fragmented local units (Johnson 1961; Key 1964). Yet there is some research suggesting that, either at the onset of World War II or during the New Deal, non-Southern Democratic state legislatures (mostly in Northern and Western Democratic states) started to shift toward a more liberal position on social issues such as civil rights and race (Feinstein and Schickler 2008). Although this gradual shift was not uniform across Democratic legislatures, Roosevelt's expansion of federal roles into state affairs triggered a transition into the nationalization of the Democratic Party policy agenda.

Historical shifts in the political ideologies of politicians, the role of government and its level of involvement in social affairs, and how ideology informs policy at the state level did not happen at the same pace and time as it happened at the federal level. At the state level, it was the Southern Democratic states that finally shifted more abruptly toward the Republican Party by the 1960s. Before the PR, the 11 states of the Confederacy were solidly controlled by Democrats, without a single partisan transition of power before the PR. Some research suggests that the nationalization of Democratic policy agendas was already complete in non-Southern states by the 1960s (Feinstein and Schickler 2008), while it was the Republican Party that most notably shifted toward conservatism in the 1960s (Valentino and Sears 2005). Although a comprehensive nationalization of both parties' policy agendas (i.e., policy agendas coordinated in a top-down, federal-state manner) did not crystallize until the 1960s, it is possible to theorize that state legislatures could have been affecting the social determinants of health prior to the PR of the 1960s, even if in a heterogeneous way relative to after the 1960s given the South/non-South dichotomy of the Democratic Party.

Racial convergence in both infant and maternal health were detected during and shortly after the civil rights movement; then the gap started to increase once again. Research reports that salutary health impacts related to the elimination of Jim Crow laws and the desegregation of hospitals were mostly detected in the South (Almond and Chay 2006; Chay and Greenstone 2000; Krieger et al. 2013). Yet the progress of efforts that originated in the civil rights movement to dismantle structural racism have continuously faced political opposition. Today we know that the civil rights movement, and the sequence of political events it ignited, were not enough to stop historically rooted socioeconomic, welfare, and public health and medical destitutions of Black people and other minorities as well as women. For example, several of the programs fostered under President Johnson were reformed under President Nixon; and, critically, Nixon's Southern Strategy—in reaction to the civil rights movement agenda—molded the new socially conservative role of race in the distribution of public goods and services, including the functioning of the US economy and capitalism (Inwood 2015).

A back-and-forth movement of policy prescription and execution was established between the parties at the national and state levels. Coded racial politics infiltrated the behavior of the electorate, bureaucracies, political actors, and institutions, affecting the ideological direction of policy. The use of a racial code in policy and social affairs marked the shift from Jim Crow or "old-fashioned" racism—focused on legalized forms of racial segregation and the explicit belief in the inherent inferiority of Black people (Sheatsley 1966)—to a more subtle yet explicitly political "symbolic racism" (Sears et al. 1997). This symbolic racism blends the perception that Black people violate traditional sociocultural American values with opposition to race-targeted (e.g., affirmative action, racial integration of schools, federal assistance to Black people) and race-neutral (e.g., privatization of health care, raising taxes, concern for the environment) policies that, directly or indirectly, differentially distribute public goods and services between the races (Chanin 2018; Sears and Henry 2003; Tesler and Sears 2010). Symbolic racism has been consistently shown to positively correlate with conservative political ideology and higher preference for the Republican Party, its policy platform, and Republican candidates, thus representing a powerful political force in deciding which officials hold office and make policy during the post-PR era (Citrin and Sears 2014; Kinder and Ryan 2017). As symbolic racism operates through political, cultural, and ideological environments that inform policy, it connects the structural components of racism that produce racial disparities in health. For example, since the 1960s, research has unsurprisingly shown that the IMR is a public health indicator exquisitely sensitive to variations in the social determinants of health that are heavily influenced by party control (Rodriguez 2019). This is especially true because the newborn and pregnant women encapsulate two periods of the human life span—for infants and women, respectively—of critical vulnerability.

As the political parties codify differential access to resources, power, and opportunity by race into policy, they also inject both practical barriers and stressors into the lives of racial-minority women and poor women of all races (Geronimus and Thompson 2004). The distribution of stressors and barriers that result from policy take the form of differential housing and food insecurity, imprisonment and segregation, social stigmas and discrimination, persistent material adversity, exposure to environmental hazards, and lack of access to high-quality medical services, among others. As social safety net resources are differentially affected by the ideological direction of policy, health outcomes of racial minorities and the poor become endogenous to whether people access resources, power, and opportunities. For example, Bound, Schoenbaum, and Waidmann (1996) report that most of the Black-white gap in labor force participation can be explained by the health differences between Blacks and whites. Similarly, Rodriguez (2018) reports that 56% of the sociopolitical participation difference between poor and nonpoor individuals can be accounted for by their differences in health. In terms of infant and maternal health, stressors and practical barriers are known to increase the prevalence of pregnancy risk factors such as maternal hypertension, obesity, and diabetes, while practical barriers decrease access to health care and technology—such as adequate responsiveness of clinicians to the needs of pregnant, laboring, and postpartum mothers of color, or access to surfactant treatments or neonatal intensive care for their newborns—that might disrupt their translation from morbidity to maternal and infant mortality (Henry-Sanchez and Geronimus 2013).

Hypotheses

The current study places the earlier results of Rodriguez and colleagues in historical context by extending the time period analyzed to cover a century, 1915–2017, rather than starting in 1965. Doing so allows us to isolate the political climates that generate ideologically opposed policy agendas attributable to partisan power, by leveraging the transformational period of the PR. At the national level, it is expected that the full combination of the abolition of Jim Crow, the civil rights movement and its traumatic events (e.g., protests, riots, assassinations, racial terror, and lynching), and the subsequent immense production of policy acts directly and indirectly related to health should generate observable partisan effects on IMRs. We thus hypothesize that different effects on infant mortality should be detectable for presidents before and after 1965—a critical year during the PR for public health law (Forgotson 1967; Rodriguez 2019; Rodriguez, Bound, and Geronimus 2014a; Rodriguez et al. 2021).

However, the policy-ideology connection and federal-state policy dynamics did not evolve at the same pace and time for the two parties. The Democratic Party started a top-down nationalization process of its policy agenda out of Southern states as a response to the Great Depression—that is, much earlier than the PR, when both parties adapted their national agendas in response to the civil rights movement, with the Republican Party now consolidating federal-state ideological and policy dynamics. Thus, we hypothesize that state IMR fluctuations will follow fluctuations in the party shifts controlling state legislatures, but the direction of such fluctuations should not shift from before to after the PR in non-Southern states.

Data and Methods

State overall and racial infant mortality data for 1941–2017 are from the Centers for Disease Control and Prevention. Vital statistics for this period are from the National Center for Health Statistics. For the period 1915–1940, the data are from Eriksson, Niemesh, and Thomasson (2018), which corrects for underregistration of births. Since Hispanic origin is not available during the early years of the study period, for consistency our racial mortality rates are for whites and Blacks including Hispanics for the majority of our study period, 1915–2014 (i.e., infant mortality data for 2015–2017 are for non-Hispanic white and Black infants). The party compositions of state legislatures are from the updated dataset in Klarner

(2013), Klarner (2003), Dubin (2007), and the National Conference of State Legislatures (table 2A, appendix).

Our data are multilevel with some variables varying by state and year (e.g., party control of state legislatures), while others vary only by year (e.g., the president's party) such that they take the same value for all observations within states. Accordingly, for each of the periods (pre-1966 and post-1965), we separately estimate the effect of the president's party using a two-stage procedure. First, we estimate the coefficients for the state-specific variables following two-way fixed effects model specification:

$$M_{st} = \beta_0 + \beta_1 L_{st} + \beta_2 U_{st} + \beta_3 (L*U)_{st} + S_s + T_t + \varepsilon_{st}. \qquad (1)$$

where M_{st} is the natural logarithm of the IMR in state s and year t. The terms L_{st} and U_{st} are one-year lagged dummy variables for party control of the lower and upper chamber of the state legislature, respectively, in state s and year t, coded "1" if the percentage of Republican representatives is higher than 50%, "0" otherwise. R_t is a 1-year lagged dummy indicating the party of the president (coded "1" if the president is Republican, "0" if Democrat). S_s are state fixed effects; T_t are year fixed effects; and ε_{st} is the error term. Our difference in difference estimates are identified off of contrasts between states that did not experience a change in party control of one or both chambers in a particular year. By including state and year fixed effects, we control for overall trends and permanent differences across states. We are, however, not controlling for unobserved differences across states that may change at roughly the same time as the party control change of state legislatures; thus, causal inferences should be made cautiously.

We recover from equation 1 the fitted coefficients ($\widehat{T_t}$) on the year dummies T_t and use them as our dependent variable in equation 2:

$$\widehat{T_t} = \delta_0 + \delta_1 R_t + f(t) + u_t. \qquad (2)$$

These coefficients on the year dummies represent the time trend of M_{st} accounting for specifications indicated in equation 1. In equation 2, $f(t)$ stands for a function of time at the national level—in this case, the Hodrick-Prescott filter function with smoothing parameter $\gamma = 100$. δ_1 provides an estimate of the effect of the president's party on M_{st} in units that are relative to trend $f(t)$. u_t is the error term. As is the case with the cross-state analysis, we are not controlling for unobserved factors that might have changed at roughly the same time as the president's party changed. Controlling for observable factors when possible—such as the unemployment rate—that change across states over time has not qualitatively altered our conclusions (Rodriguez, Bound, and Geronimus 2014a, 2014b; Rodriguez et al. 2021).

The two equations are estimated using OLS, and the standard errors are estimated using the Newey-West estimator (panel-corrected in equation 1), which is robust to arbitrary patterns of serial correlation. The literature has established that in finite samples the Newey-West estimator tends to underestimate sampling variability (Jansson 2004). To account for this, the 95% confidence intervals and *p* values were adjusted using fixed-beta asymptotics (Kiefer and Vogelsang 2005; Vogelsang 2012). The distribution of the error terms is assumed heteroskedastic and autocorrelated up to a lag of four years (the period of a president's and a state representative's term). Equation 1 is estimated using state-level time-constant weights, where these weights correspond to annual state shares of living births respectively (such that $\sum w_s = 1$ in any given year) and then averaged for states across all years.

Four states were excluded from the analytic sample (Nebraska because of a unicameral system; Alaska and Hawaii because they became states in 1959; and Minnesota, which had a "nonpartisan era" most notably during the pre-1966 period). Also, not all states reported Black IMRs during the study period, and many others showed very low numbers of Black infant deaths (<20) as a result of a very small Black population, which did not allow for reliable estimates of the IMR. For these reasons, we included 31 states in our race-specific analyses (table 3A, appendix).

Results

Figure 1 displays trends for race-specific mean IMRs of Southern (defined in terms of states that participated in the Confederacy) and non-Southern states, with the vertical scales in natural logarithm units. The figure covers the period 1927 to 2017, when the unbalanced panel data are least pronounced. Figure 1 shows that IMRs fell dramatically over the last century, with slowdowns in their decline during the civil rights movement period and then during the last two decades of our study period. In the early period, a large part of the decline can be attributed to public health measures, while in the later period developments in medicine play a central role. Distressingly, during the last half century, the racial gap in IMR has widened (figure 2).

Figure 3 shows the distribution of years of Democratic control of the upper and lower chambers across states. Although there are numerous shifts in partisan control across states during the post-PR period, this was

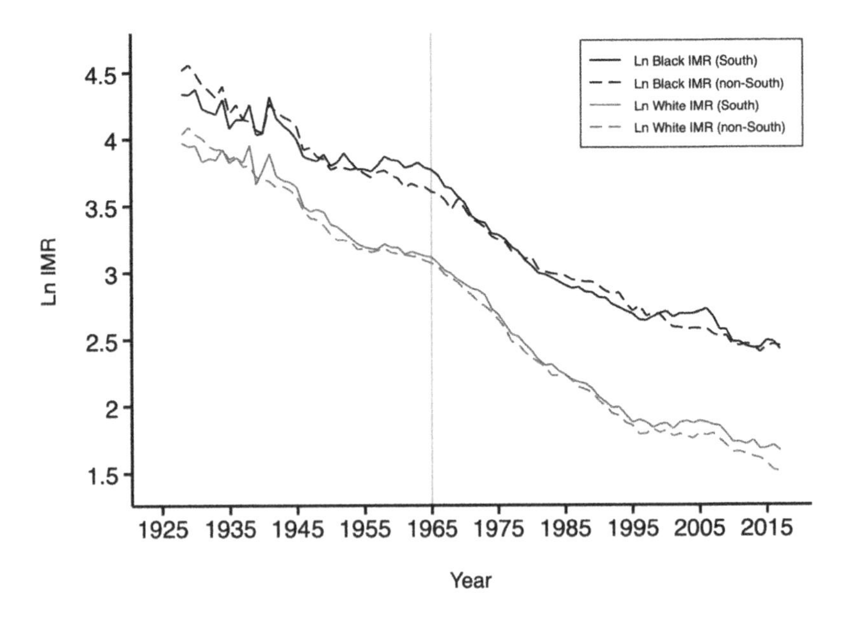

Figure 1 IMR trends in Southern and non-Southern states, by race.

not the case in the South before the PR. This is critical because our identification strategy relies on partisan shifts occurring between and within states, a condition that is only partially met during the pre-PR period. In particular, the lower and upper chambers in the 11 Southern states of the Confederacy were solidly controlled by Democrats, with not a single partisan transition happening in these states before the PR. Accordingly, Southern states are not contributing to the partisan IMR difference estimates specified in equation 1 for the pre-PR period. This is central for the interpretation of our results: partisan differences in IMRs captured by our estimates in the pre-PR period are, therefore, exclusive for party dynamics that occurred out of Southern states.

Table 1 shows the parameter estimates from the two-stage procedure. The upper panel reports results for the pre-PR period, whereas the bottom panel reports results for the post-PR period. Results are organized from left to right for overall, white, and Black IMRs, respectively, and by sample. For each dependent variable, models to the left do not include an interactive term between party control in the lower and upper chambers—that is, when the state legislature is controlled by Republicans. Models to the right include the interactive term. These are the models we will use for interpretation of results. Estimates of β_1 in equation 1 represent estimates

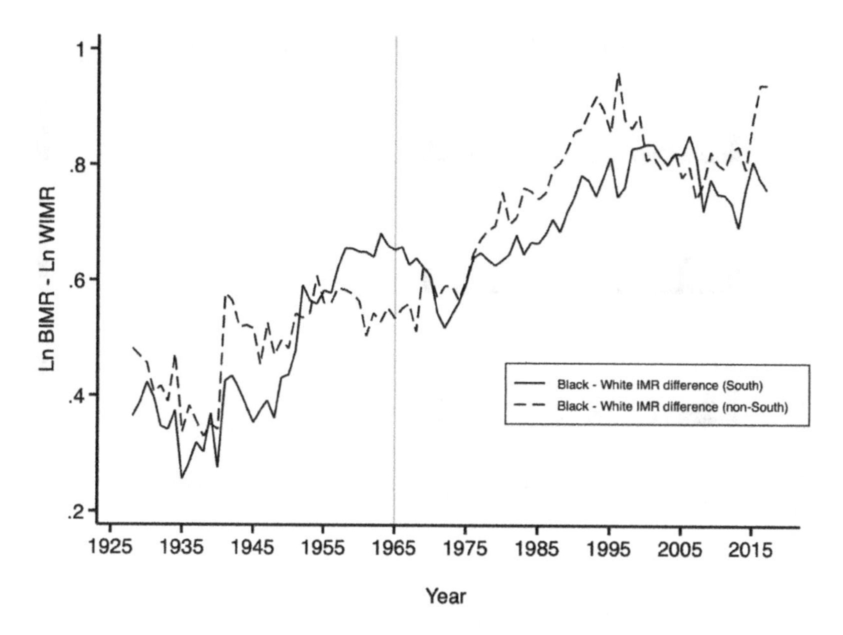

Figure 2 Racial difference IMR trends in Southern and non-Southern states.

of the average, net of trend, difference in log infant mortality associated with a transition within a state between a situation where both chambers of the legislature are under Democratic control to one in which the lower chamber is in Republican control. Estimates of β_2 represent comparable estimates for the upper chamber. Within-state transitions between complete control of the legislature by Democrats to complete control by Republicans are represented by $\beta_1+\beta_2+\beta_3$.

Pre-PR estimates for state legislatures in table 1 show that, net of trend, states with legislatures under complete Republican control experience higher IMRs than do states under Democratic control. Thus, for example, in the 46-state sample, the transition from Democratic- to Republican-controlled legislatures is associated with a net-of-trend increase in IMR of 6.9% (=.116 - .043 - .004) ($p<.001$). In contrast, the estimates imply shifts from a Democratic-controlled legislature to one with Republican control of only one of the two chambers are not associated with statistically significant changes in the IMR. This pattern persists across the samples that include overall (i.e., total) births and white births. In contrast, the estimates in column 10 suggest that for Black infants, it is control of the lower chamber that matters. Additionally, these estimates suggest that party control has more of an effect on IMR for Black infants than for

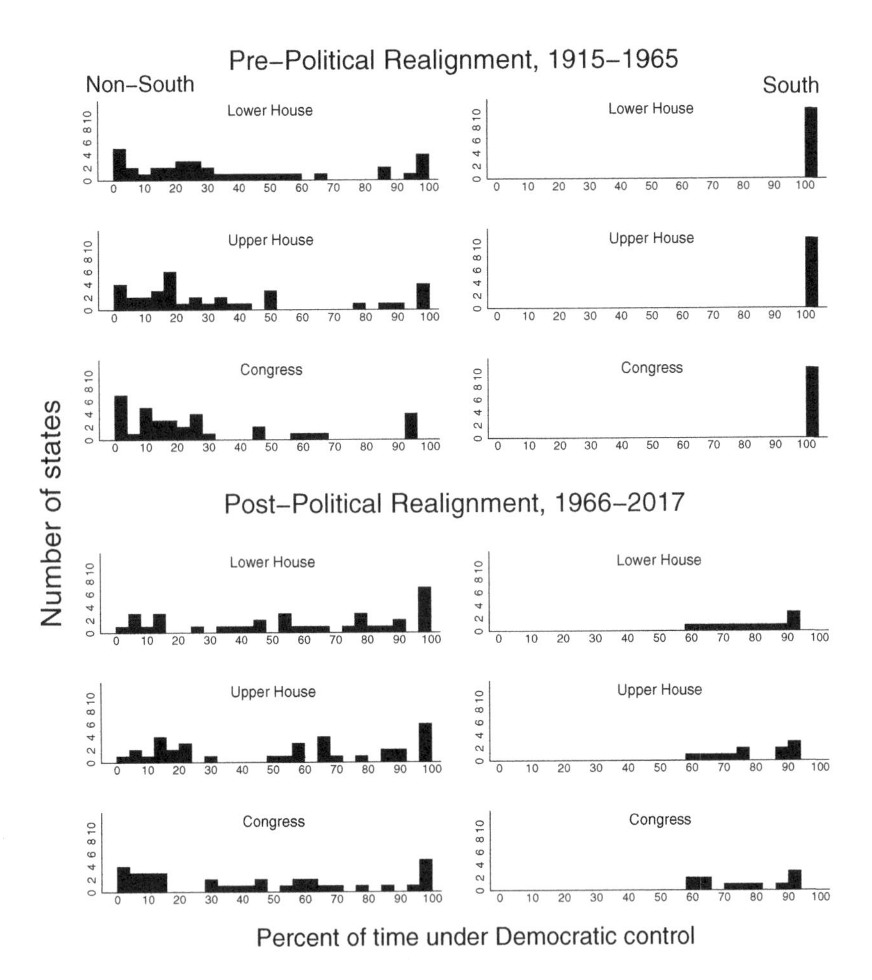

Figure 3 Percentage of time under Democratic control in state legislatures, 1915–2017.

white infants (for example, $\hat{\beta}_1+\hat{\beta}_2+\hat{\beta}_3=.108$ [$p < .001$] in column 10, while it is .028 [$p<.1$] in column 8).

We emphasize that these estimates represent averages across states that experienced transitions in control of the lower chamber, the upper chamber, or both. During this period of time, Southern states were under the control of the Democratic Party and do not contribute to these estimates. In the post-PR period, when both state legislature chambers are under Republican control there are independent detrimental effects on IMR (estimates of β_1 and β_2 in equation 1). During the post-PR period party control estimates for Blacks and whites are roughly comparable.

Table 1 Parameter Estimates for Presidential Party (Republican) and Party Control of State Legislature (Republican) Effects on State Overall and Race-Specific IMRs before and after the PR, 1915–2017

		Before PR (1915–1965)									
		Ln IMR (46 states)		Ln IMR (31 states)		Ln WIMR (46 states)		Ln WIMR (31 states)		Ln BIMR (31 states)	
		(1)	(2)	(3)	(4)	(5)	(6)	(7)	(8)	(9)	(10)
Lower chamber	Coeff.	.025	−.043	.030	−.040	.013	−.011	.013	−.010	.096	.081
	95% CI	±.037	±.058	±.040	±.060	±.022	±.033	±.023	±.036	±.050	±.073
	p	.179	.150	.145	.195	.244	.501	.275	.581	.000	.031
Upper chamber	Coeff.	.063	−.004	.071	−.002	.012	−.013	.021	−.004	.018	−.001
	95% CI	±.048	±.034	±.053	±.040	±.024	±.027	±.026	±.030	±.059	±.066
	p	.011	.810	.008	.937	.308	.345	.099	.773	.565	.980
Lower x upper	Coeff.		.116		.120		.043		.042		.028
	95% CI		±.069		±.071		±.043		±.045		±.091
	p		.001		.001		.044		.071		.540
President	Coeff.	−.007	−.005	−.007	−.005	−.009	−.008	−.008	−.008	−.009	−.009
	95% CI	±.017	±.017	±.018	±.018	±.017	±.017	±.016	±.017	±.032	±.032
	p	.439	.543	.461	.572	.305	.332	.320	.351	.574	.579
Joint test	Chi-2	11.88	16.59	12.23	16.61	3.70	6.84	5.72	7.27	19.76	19.95
	p	.003	.001	.002	.001	.157	.077	.057	.064	.000	.000

(continued)

Table 1 Parameter Estimates for Presidential Party (Republican) and Party Control of State Legislature (Republican) Effects on State Overall and Race-Specific IMRs before and after the PR, 1915–2017 *(continued)*

		After PR (1966–2017)									
		Ln IMR (46 states)		Ln IMR (31 states)		Ln WIMR (46 states)		Ln WIMR (31 states)		Ln BIMR (31 states)	
		(1)	(2)	(3)	(4)	(5)	(6)	(7)	(8)	(9)	(10)
Lower chamber	Coeff.	.032	.042	.032	.040	.022	.028	.021	.024	.032	.054
	95% CI	±.018	±.025	±.020	±.030	±.016	±.021	±.018	±.025	±.027	±.035
	p	.001	.001	.003	.008	.007	.009	.018	.052	.024	.003
Upper chamber	Coeff.	.022	.027	.028	.031	.024	.027	.031	.032	.007	.017
	95% CI	±.021	±.025	±.023	±.027	±.017	±.021	±.018	±.022	±.031	±.035
	p	.035	.035	.018	.022	.005	.011	.001	.004	.637	.343
Lower x upper	Coeff.		−.015		−.012		−.009		−.004		−.033
	95% CI		±.030		±.034		±.027		±.029		±.043
	p		.333		.484		.509		.778		.132
President	Coeff.	.018	.018	.018	.018	.021	.021	.021	.021	.021	.021
	95% CI	±.011	±.011	±.011	±.011	±.011	±.011	±.011	±.011	±.018	±.018
	p	.001	.001	.002	.002	.000	.000	.000	.000	.024	.023
Joint test	Chi-2	21.8	22.53	21.24	21.57	23.44	23.72	24.94	25.01	6.37	9.96
	p	.000	.000	.000	.000	.000	.000	.000	.000	.041	.019

Notes: *P* computed from Newey-West panel-corrected standard errors using fixed-bandwith asymptotics. Panel error structure is assumed heteroskedastic and autocorrelated up to a lag of four years. Regressions weighted using time-constant averaged number of overall or race-specific births. All states included with the exception of Nebraska, Alaska, Hawaii, and Minnesota (n = 46). The "31" states are the 31 states with a Black population large enough to retrieve reliable mortality rates for Black infants (table 3A, appendix). State legislature estimates are from equation 1; presidential party effects are from equation 2. The joint test tests for the statistical significance of all party control of state legislatures terms in equation 1 ($\beta_1 = \beta_2 = 0$ in odd columns, and $\beta_1 = \beta_2 = \beta_3 = 0$ in even columns).

Table 1 also shows that, in all instances, overall and race-specific IMRs are, net of trend, lower under Republican presidents before the PR, although these estimates are imprecisely estimated (estimates of δ_1 in equation 2). This lack of precision, is, perhaps, not too surprising. There were relatively few party transitions in presidential power during the 1915–1965 period, and there were massive, potentially confounding effects (two world wars, a pandemic, multiple severe recessions, and the Great Depression). Presidential estimates for the post-PR period are more precisely estimated (the confidence intervals for the earlier period are more than 50% wider than for the later period), showing that overall and race-specific IMRs are, net of trend, about 2% higher during Republican administrations relative to Democratic ones ($p < 0.05$). The magnitudes of the presidential estimates are similar for Black and white IMRs. The magnitudes of Republican-controlled state legislatures are larger than those of Republican presidents in both periods. That the direction and importance of presidents consistently shift from before to after the PR whereas they do not shift for state legislatures supports our hypothesis.

Discussion

We used a historical framework to construe the connections between the racialization of policy and the ideological direction of policy agendas imparted by the political parties and their elected officials. Findings show that, net of trend, overall and race-specific IMRs were higher under the more racially conservative party, before and after the PR, respectively. These patterns were detected for the institutional arrangements—executive or legislative, national or state—that allow parties to execute a racially conservative agenda. In this sense, population health in the United States follows partisan cycles, and it is politicized by means of racialized policy (Michener 2019; Michener and Brower 2020). We also found that the partisan differences in IMRs from before to after the PR are large and generally statistically significant. Whether this means that the role of the two parties in maintaining health inequity actually reversed, or whether it means the racialized underpinnings of the New Deal (for state governments) and the PR of the 1960s (at the national level) created a fundamentally new relationship between the president's party, state legislatures, and pregnancy outcomes, our findings underscore the political mutability of population inequities in health.

Although the majority of the variation in IMRs belongs to low-frequency variation—that is, to historical factors that were removed from our estimates—the effects we detect are substantial. Our estimates represent annual average partisan differences in IMRs between pre- and post-PR periods (table 1). To put the size of our estimates in context, in their studies of the effects of Medicaid on IMR, Currie and Gruber (1996) and Goodman-Bacon (2018) report that the increase in Medicaid eligibility of pregnant women during the introductory years of the program was associated with a total 7% (1979–1990) and 8% (1965–1980) decline in IMR, respectively. These estimates are comparable in magnitude to our estimates of the impact that the shift in the partisan control of a state legislature would have on IMRs (table 1).

Our results also show that IMRs are not only influenced by national partisan politics but also by partisan control of state legislatures. Although there is some variation in our state legislature estimates, these were, overall, higher than those detected for presidents in both periods (table 1). We also find some consistency in the partisan-ideological direction of this association, as some research suggests that Democratic states started to move toward less conservative stances relative to Republican states as the result of Roosevelt's nationalization efforts to counteract the effects of the Great Depression (Feinstein and Schickler 2008; Hopkins, Schickler, and Azizi 2021). These findings confirm and update recent analyses showing the importance of national unified government (Torche and Rauf 2021) and, more explicitly, state legislatures, for public health policy and their effects on population health, including infant health (Rodriguez et al. 2021; Torche and Rauf 2021). Research covering periods after the PR suggests that state-level effects of conservative policy are expected, especially after the 1970s, during the "New Federalism" period (Montez 2019; Montez 2020; Montez et al. 2020; Montez, Hayward, and Zajacova 2019). Our findings show that political state-level effects have been present since much earlier, including at least part of the first half of the 20th century.

We note particular limitations in our study. Although we use panel data corrected for underregistration of births (Eriksson, Niemesh, and Thomasson 2018), our panel data estimates are crude. Data scarcity, especially for the pre-PR period, precluded us from adding controls beyond time and state fixed effects in our models. Key data sources like the Current Population Survey became large in scale and reliable only after World War II. However, in national-level analyses for which controls were available (not presented here), especially for the post-PR period, they did not change the results of our analyses.

Research is inconclusive about specific nationalization and ideological shift periods in state legislatures before the PR. Lack of variation in party control of state legislatures (especially in the South) and of the presidency (the Franklin Roosevelt and Truman administrations covered 20 years of Democratic presidents) in the pre-PR period precluded us from expanding our model specifications. Even though our analysis presents a first approximation of federalism's effects on health during the last century, further analysis on how the ideology-policy connection and federal-state policy agendas affect health is warranted.

Overall, our findings are important considering that the United States has had a very stable two-party system during the last century. As the two parties naturally promote policy agendas that make it easier for voters, lobbies, and stakeholders to differentiate them, a conservative dimension of policy is an unavoidable component of government activity. Socially conservative policy making, governance, and the enforcement of the rule of law that weaken the welfare system and consequently the social determinants of health are entrenched in the historical balance of power that fluctuates between the parties, nationally and at the state level. Our findings support the notion that one important answer to how socially conservative politics in the United States ended up requiring policies that undermine welfare systems to be conservative is structural racism. If health disparities are entrenched in spite of an enormous production of scientific discoveries and their resulting policy solutions and intervention designs, it is because those policies and interventions have been racialized by the governmental apparatus, too. We have arrived at a point in time where promoting health equity requires us to identify how we can change US politics and its racialized nature.

▪ ▪ ▪

Javier M. Rodríguez is an associate professor of politics and government and codirector of both the Inequality and Policy Research Center and the Institute for Democratic Renewal at Claremont Graduate University. After receiving his PhD from UCLA, he completed his postdoctoral training at the Population Studies Center of the University of Michigan. His research is published in a number of multidisciplinary journals, including *International Journal of Epidemiology, Health Affairs*, and *Social Science and Medicine*. He has recently been awarded research grants from the Russell Sage Foundation, the Social Security Administration, and the National Institute on Aging.
javier.rodriguez@cgu.edu

Byengseon Bae is a PhD student in political science at Claremont Graduate University, where he studies American politics and political philosophy.

Arline T. Geronimus is a professor with the Department of Health Behavior and Health Education at the University of Michigan and a research professor at the Population Studies Center of the Institute for Social Research, where she also is the founding director of the Public Health Demography training program. She is affiliated with the Center for Research on Ethnicity, Culture, and Health, and she is an elected member of the Institute of Medicine of the National Academies of Science.

John Bound is a professor with the Department of Economics at the University of Michigan and a research professor at the Population Studies Center of the Institute for Social Research, where he is the director of the Michigan Center for the Demography of Aging. He is a faculty associate at the National Bureau of Economic Research, where he is affiliated with the Labor Studies Program and the Education and Aging Program. He is an elected fellow of the Econometric Society and the Society for Labor Economists.

References

Aldrich, John H. 1995. *Why Parties? The Origin and Transformation of Political Parties in America*. Chicago: University of Chicago Press.

Almond, Douglas, and Kenneth Y. Chay. 2006. "The Long-Run and Intergenerational Impact of Poor Infant Health: Evidence from Cohorts Born During the Civil Rights Era." Unpublished manuscript, February. users.nber.org/~almond/chay_npc_paper.pdf.

Bartels, Larry M., and Katherine J. Cramer. 2019. "The Struggle(s) for Equality: Civil Rights, Women's Rights, and Political Climate." Paper presented at the Annual Meeting of the American Political Science Association, Washington Hilton, Washington, DC, August 29.

Beck, Paul A. 1974. "A Socialization Theory of Party Realignment." In *The Politics of Future Citizens*, edited by Richard G. Niemi, 199–219. San Francisco: Jossey-Bass.

Bhatia, Amiya, Nancy Krieger, and S. V. Subramanian. 2019. "Learning from History about Reducing Infant Mortality: Contrasting the Centrality of Structural Interventions to Early 20th-Century Successes in the United States to Their Neglect in Current Global Initiatives." *Milbank Quarterly* 97, no. 1: 285–345.

Bonilla-Silva, Eduardo. 2006. *Racism without Racists: Color-Blind Racism and the Persistence of Racial Inequality in the United States*. 2nd ed. Lanham, MD: Rowman and Littlefield.

Bound, John, Michael Schoenbaum, and Timothy Waidmann. 1996. "Race Differences in Labor Force Attachment and Disability Status." *Gerontologist* 36, no. 3: 311–21.

Brennan, Mary C. 1995. *Turning Right in the Sixties : The Conservative Capture of the GOP*. Chapel Hill: University of North Carolina Press.

Burnham, Walter D. 1970. *Critical Elections and the Mainsprings of American Politics*. New York: W. W. Norton and Company.

Burnham, Walter D. 1975. "Party Systems and the Political Process." In *The American Party Systems: Stages of Political Development*, edited by William N. Chambers, 227–307. New York: Oxford University Press.

Carmines, Edward G., and James A. Stimson. 1989. *Issue Evolution: Race and the Transformation of American Politics*. Princeton, NJ: Princeton University Press.

Caughey, Devin. 2018. *The Unsolid South: Mass Politics and National Representation in a One-Party Enclave*. Princeton, NJ: Princeton University Press.

Chanin, Jesse. 2018. "The Effect of Symbolic Racism on Environmental Concern and Environmental Action." *Environmental Sociology* 4, no. 4: 457–69.

Chay, Kenneth Y., and Michael Greenstone. 2000. "The Convergence in Black-White Infant Mortality Rates during the 1960s." *American Economic Review* 90, no. 2: 326–32.

Citrin, Jack, and David O. Sears. 2014. *American Identity and the Politics of Multiculturalism*. New York: Cambridge University Press.

Clubb, Jerome M., William H. Flanigan, and Nancy H. Zingale. 1980. *Partisan Realignment: Voters, Parties, and Government in American History*. Beverly Hills, CA: Sage Publications.

Cottrell, David, Michael C. Herron, Javier M. Rodriguez, and Daniel A. Smith. 2019. "Mortality, Incarceration, and African American Disenfranchisement in the Contemporary United States." *American Politics Research* 47, no. 2: 195–237.

Currie, Janet, and Jonathan Gruber. 1996. "Saving Babies: The Efficacy and Cost of Recent Changes in the Medicaid Eligibility of Pregnant Women." *Journal of Political Economy* 104, no. 6: 1263–96.

Dubin, Michael J. 2007. *Party Affiliations in the State Legislatures: A Year by Year Summary, 1796–2006*. Jefferson, NC: McFarland and Company.

Eriksson, Katherine, Gregory T. Niemesh, and Melissa Thomasson. 2018. "Revising Infant Mortality Rates for the Early Twentieth Century United States." *Demography* 55, no. 6: 2001–24.

Ertel, Karen A., Tamarra James-Todd, Kenneth Kleinman, Nancy Krieger, Matthew Gillman, Rosalind Wright, and Janet Rich-Edwards. 2012. "Racial Discrimination, Response to Unfair Treatment, and Depressive Symptoms among Pregnant Black and African American Women in the United States." *Annals of Epidemiology* 22, no. 12: 840–46.

Feinstein, Brian D., and Eric Schickler. 2008. "Platforms and Partners: The Civil Rights Realignment Reconsidered." *Studies in American Political Development* 22, no. 1: 1–31.

Forgotson, Edward H. 1967. "1965: The Turning Point in Health Law—1966 Reflections." *American Journal of Public Health and the Nation's Health* 57, no. 6: 934–46.

Geronimus, Arline T. 1992. "The Weathering Hypothesis and the Health of African-American Women and Infants: Evidence and Speculations." *Ethnicity and Disease* 2, no. 3: 207–21.

Geronimus, Arline T. 2000. "To Mitigate, Resist, or Undo: Addressing Structural Influences on the Health of Urban Populations." *American Journal of Public Health* 90, no. 6: 867–72.

Geronimus, Arline T., and J. Phillip Thompson. 2004. "To Denigrate, Ignore, or Disrupt: Racial Inequality in Health and the Impact of a Policy-Induced Breakdown of African American Communities." *Du Bois Review* 1, no. 2: 247–79.

Gerring, John E. 1998. *Party Ideologies in America, 1828–1996*. Cambridge, UK: Cambridge University Press.

Goodman-Bacon, Andrew. 2018. "Public Insurance and Mortality: Evidence from Medicaid Implementation." *Journal of Political Economy* 126, no. 1: 216–62.

Green, Donald P., Bradley Palmquist, and Eric Schickler. 2002. *Partisan Hearts and Minds : Political Parties and the Social Identities of Voters*. New Haven, CT: Yale University Press.

Heersink, Boris, and Jeffery A. Jenkins. 2020. *Republican Party Politics and the American South, 1865–1968*. Cambridge: Cambridge University Press.

Henry-Sanchez, Brenda L., and Arline T. Geronimus. 2013. "Racial/Ethnic Disparities in Infant Mortality among US Latinos." *Du Bois Review* 10, no. 1: 205–31.

Hopkins, Daniel J., Eric Schickler, and David Azizi. 2021. "From Many Divides, One? The Polarization and Nationalization of American State Party Platforms, 1918–2017." *SSRN*, March 15. papers.ssrn.com/sol3/papers.cfm?abstract_id=3772946.

Inwood, Joshua F. J. 2015. "Neoliberal Racism: The 'Southern Strategy' and the Expanding Geographies of White Supremacy." *Social and Cultural Geography* 16, no. 4: 407–23.

Jansson, Michael. 2004. "The Error in Rejection Probability of Simple Autocorrelation Robust Tests." *Econometrica* 72, no. 3: 937–46.

Johnson, Claudius O. 1961. *American State and Local Government*. 3rd ed. New York: Thomas Y. Crowell and Company.

Key, V. O., Jr. 1955. "A Theory of Critical Elections." *Journal of Politics* 17, no. 1: 3–18.

Key, V. O., Jr. 1964. *Politics, Parties, and Pressure Groups*. New York: Thomas Y. Crowell and Company.

KFF (Kaiser Family Foundation). 2011. "Timeline: History of Health Reform in the US." www.kff.org/wp-content/uploads/2011/03/5-02-13-history-of-health-reform .pdf (accessed October 20, 2021).

Kiefer, Nicholas M., and Timothy J. Vogelsang. 2005. "A New Asymptotic Theory for Heteroskedasticity-Autocorrelation Robust Tests." *Econometric Theory* 21, no. 6: 1130–64.

Kinder, Donald R., and Timothy J. Ryan. 2017. "Prejudice and Politics Re-Examined: The Political Significance of Implicit Racial Bias." *Political Science Research and Methods* 5, no. 2: 241–59.

Klarner, Carl. 2003. "The Measurement of the Partisan Balance of State Government." *State Politics and Policy Quarterly* 3, no. 3: 309–19.

Klarner, Carl. 2013. "State Partisan Balance Data, 1937–2011." Harvard Dataverse. doi.org/10.7910/DVN/LZHMG3 (accessed October 20, 2021).

Krieger, Nancy, Jarvis T. Chen, Brent Coull, Pamela D. Waterman, and Jason Beckfield. 2013. "The Unique Impact of Abolition of Jim Crow Laws on Reducing Inequities in Infant Death Rates and Implications for Choice of Comparison Groups in Analyzing Societal Determinants of Health." *American Journal of Public Health* 103, no. 12: 2234–44.

Levendusky, Matthew. 2009. *The Partisan Sort: How Liberals Became Democrats and Conservatives Became Republicans*. Chicago: University of Chicago Press.

Michener, Jamila. 2019. "Policy Feedback in a Racialized Polity." *Policy Studies Journal* 47, no. 2: 423–50.

Michener, Jamila, and Margaret T. Brower. 2020. "What's Policy Got to Do with It? Race, Gender, and Economic Inequality in the United States." *Daedalus* 149, no. 1: 100–18.

Mickey, Robert W. 2008. "The Beginning of the End for Authoritarian Rule in America: Smith v. Allwright and the Abolition of the White Primary in the Deep South, 1944–1948." *Studies in American Political Development* 22, no. 2: 143–82.

Mickey, Robert W. 2015. *Paths Out of Dixie: The Democratization of Authoritarian Enclaves in America's Deep South, 1944–1972*. Princeton, NJ: Princeton University Press.

Montez, Jennifer K. 2019. "Policy Polarization and Death in the United States." *Temple Law Review* 92, no. 4: 889–916.

Montez, Jennifer K. 2020. "US State Polarization, Policymaking Power, and Population Health." *Milbank Quarterly*, October 20. doi.org/10.1111/1468-0009.12482.

Montez, Jennifer K., Jason Beckfield, Julene K. Cooney, Jacob M. Grumbach, Mark D. Hayward, Huseyin Z. Koytak, Steven H. Woolf, and Anna Zajacova. 2020. "US State Policies, Politics, and Life Expectancy." *Milbank Quarterly* 98, no. 3: 668–99.

Montez, Jennifer Karas, Mark D. Hayward, and Anna Zajacova. 2019. "Educational Disparities in Adult Health: US States as Institutional Actors on the Association." *Socius: Sociological Research for a Dynamic World*, January. doi.org/10.1177/2378023119835345.

Osborne, Danny, David O. Sears, and Nicholas A. Valentino. 2011. "The End of the Solidly Democratic South: The Impressionable-Years Hypothesis." *Political Psychology* 32, no. 1: 81–107.

Phillips, Kevin P. 1970. "The Future of American Politics." *Modern Age* 14, no. 3: 305–12.

Rodriguez, Javier M. 2018. "Health Disparities, Politics, and the Maintenance of the Status Quo: A New Theory of Inequality." *Social Science and Medicine* 200: 36–43.

Rodriguez, Javier M. 2019. "The Politics Hypothesis and Racial Disparities in Infants' Health in the United States." *SSM—Population Health*, July 6. doi.org/10.1016/j.ssmph.2019.100440.

Rodriguez, Javier M., John Bound, and Arline T. Geronimus. 2014a. "US Infant Mortality and the President's Party." *International Journal of Epidemiology* 43, no. 3: 818–26.

Rodriguez, Javier M., John Bound, and Arline T. Geronimus. 2014b. "Rejoinder: Time Series Analysis and US Infant Mortality: De-trending the Empirical from the Polemical in Political Epidemiology." *International Journal of Epidemiology* 43, no. 3: 831–34.

Rodriguez, Javier M., Arline T. Geronimus, John Bound, Rixin Wen, and Christina M. Kinane. 2021. "Partisan Control of US State Governments: Politics as a Social Determinant of Infant Health." *American Journal of Preventive Medicine*, August 23. doi.org/10.1016/j.amepre.2021.06.007.

Sears, David O., and P. J. Henry. 2003. "The Origins of Symbolic Racism." *Journal of Personality and Social Psychology* 85, no. 2: 259–75.

Sears, David O., Colette Van Laar, Mary Carrillo, and Rick Kosterman. 1997. "Is It Really Racism? The Origins of White Americans' Opposition to Race-Targeted Policies." *Public Opinion Quarterly* 61, no. 1: 16–53.

Sheatsley, Paul B. 1966. "White Attitudes toward the Negro." *Daedalus* 95, no.1: 217–38.

Tesler, Michael. 2016. *Post-Racial or Most-Racial? Race and Politics in the Obama Era*. Chicago: University of Chicago Press.

Tesler, Michael, and David O. Sears. 2010. *Obama's Race: The 2008 Election and the Dream of a Post-Racial America*. Chicago: University of Chicago Press.

Torche, Florencia, and Tamkinat Rauf. 2021. "The Political Context and Infant Health in the United States." *American Sociological Review* 86, no. 3: 377–405.

Valentino, Nicholas A., and David O. Sears. 2005. "Old Times There Are Not Forgotten: Race and Partisan Realignment in the Contemporary South." *American Journal of Political Science* 49, no. 3: 672–88.

Vogelsang, Timothy J. 2012. "Heteroskedasticity, Autocorrelation, and Spatial Correlation: Robust Inference in Linear Panel Models with Fixed-Effects." *Journal of Econometrics* 166, no. 2: 303–19.

WHO (World Health Organization). 2008. "Closing the Gap in a Generation: Health Equity through Action on the Social Determinants of Health—Final Report of the Commission on Social Determinants of Health." August 27. www.who.int/publications/i/item/WHO-IER-CSDH-08.1.

Williams, David R. 2002. "Racial/Ethnic Variations in Women's Health: The Social Embeddedness of Health." *American Journal of Public Health* 92, no. 4: 588–97.

State Policies, Racial Disparities, and Income Support: A Way to Address Infant Outcomes and the Persistent Black-White Gap?

Jessica Pearlman
Dean E. Robinson
University of Massachusetts Amherst

Abstract Low birth weight and preterm births vary by state, and Black mothers typically face twice the risk that their white counterparts do. This gap reflects an accumulation of psychosocial and material exposures that include interpersonal racism, differential experience with area-level deprivation such as residential segregation, and other harmful exposures that the authors refer to as "institutional" or "structural" racism. The authors use logistic regression models and a dataset that includes all births from 1994 to 2017 as well as five state policies from this period—Aid to Families with Dependent Children/Temporary Aid for Needy Families, housing assistance, Medicaid, minimum wage, and the earned income tax credit (EITC)—to examine whether these state social policies, designed to provide a financial safety net, are associated with risk reduction of low birth weight and preterm birth to Black and white mothers, and whether variations in state generosity attenuate the racial inequalities in birth outcomes. The authors also examine whether the relationship between state policies and racial inequalities in birth outcomes is moderated by the education level of the mother. We find that the EITC reduces the risk of low birth weight and preterm birth for Black mothers. The impact is much less consistent for white mothers. For both Black and white mothers, the benefits to birth outcomes are larger for mothers with less education.

Keywords state social policies, preterm birth, low birth weight, racism, earned income tax credit

In the United States, Black-white gaps in birth weight and preterm birth are a persistent and tragic feature of a political and economic system that produces and reproduces health inequities—differences in health outcomes that are avoidable and preventable and are therefore unjust (Whitehead

Journal of Health Politics, Policy and Law, Vol. 47, No. 2, April 2022
DOI 10.1215/03616878-9517205

1992). Black mothers have a nearly twofold greater risk of low birth weight (infants born <2500 g) and preterm birth (infants born before 37 weeks of gestation) compared to whites (Collins et al. 2000; Rosenthal and Lobel 2011). Even with comparable levels of formal education, Black women face greater risk, and the most highly educated Black mothers have higher levels of preterm and low-birth-weight infants than white mothers with the least amount of education.

While the causes of preterm birth and low birth weight are not fully understood, they are thought to reflect a complex interaction of the mother's age; genetic factors; behavioral factors, especially smoking and substance abuse; and (lack of) prenatal care. Figure 1 shows that for both outcomes, there is a graded pattern for Black and white women according to levels of educational attainment. This is consistent in analyses that examine socioeconomic statistics at the individual and area levels (Blumenshine et al. 2010). However, as noted before, at comparable points along the socioeconomic ladder, Black infants are at a higher risk (McGrady et al. 1992). The Black-white gap in infant outcomes *does not reflect mysteries of DNA*, but rather the cumulative effects of racism.[1] "Black" identity is not a discrete genetic category that captures a unique profile of medical risk but rather *a lived, contingent, and contextual experience*, which, at comparable points along the socioeconomic ladder, typically means having less access to the types of resources that promote health and more harmful psychosocial and material exposure.

Both racial (ethnic) and class inequalities thus matter to health outcomes, as these categories are "mutually constitutive" (Kawachi, Daniels, and Robinson 2005). Essentialist notions of a Black identity (or "African" or "Negro" in earlier periods) originated and evolved as ideological justification of US slavery and, in the post-Reconstruction and post–Jim Crow eras, as rationale for systems of low-wage, exploitative labor regimes (Fields 1990; Smedley 2012).

Studies of Black-white inequalities in birth outcomes in the United States have increasingly pursued analyses at two levels, starting with an assessment of risk factors for mothers (age, education, smoking, access to prenatal care, etc.) while also considering the context of racism (interpersonal and structural) in which births happen. David and Collins (1997, 2007) advanced this perspective in an important set of articles that challenged

1. For the purpose of the article, we understand "racism" to mean exposure to interpersonal, discriminatory treatment (Alhusen et al. 2016), as well as exposure to patterns of disadvantage that result in disproportionately higher levels of poverty, greater levels of unemployment, and residential segregation. In their influential book *Black Power*, Carmichael and Hamilton (1967) called this "institutional racism." We take this to be synonymous with "structural racism."

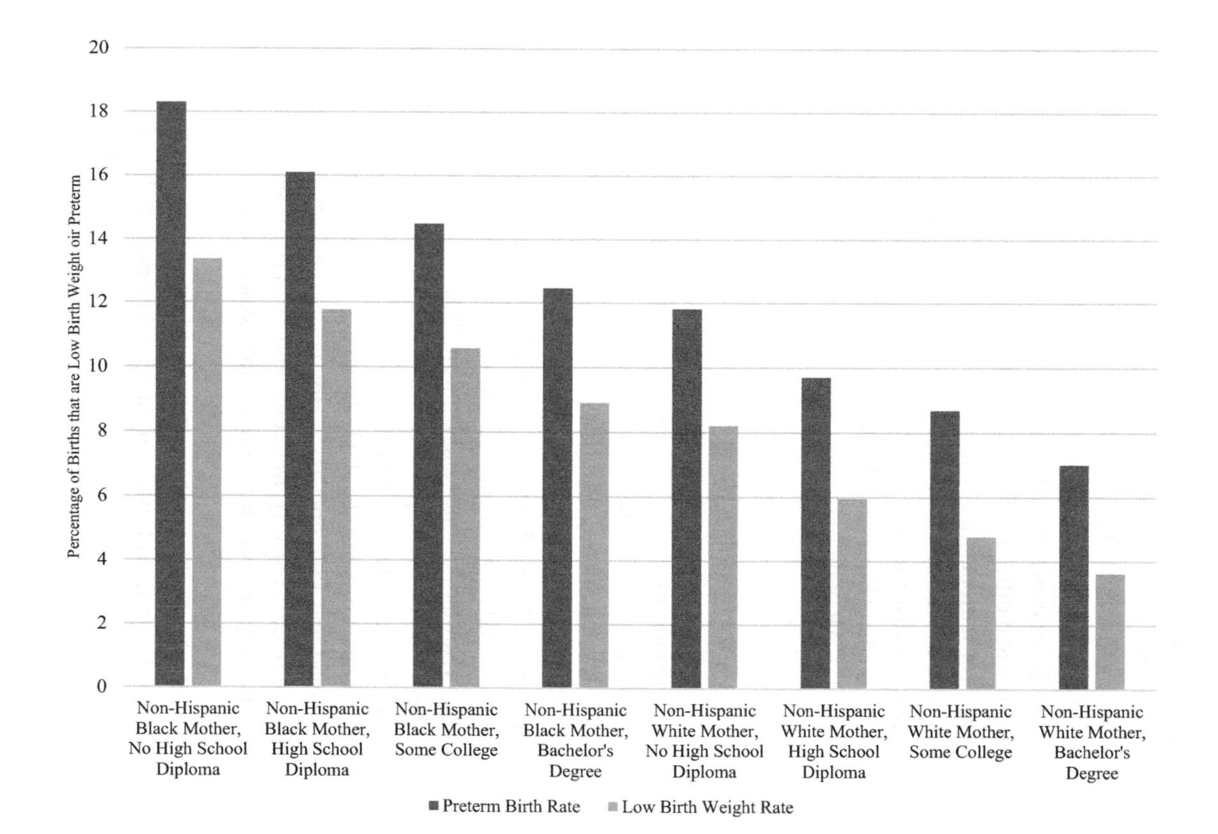

Figure 1 Low birth weight and preterm birth rates (1994–2017) by mother's race and education.

the genetic interpretation of Black-white disparities in birth outcomes by showing evidence that perceived discrimination predicted low birth weight. Subsequent studies have analyzed exposure to interpersonal discrimination in different domains, and many find an association with perceived racism that, over time, affects birth outcomes.[2]

By looking at individual-level risk factors in the context of neighborhoods or other geopolitical units of analysis, researchers have found that different metrics of concentrated disadvantage, or "deprivation," matter to birth outcomes and differ for Black and white women. Residential segregation, local (or national) labor markets, poverty rates, environmental exposures such as lead and air pollution, and racial attitudes are all associated with racial disparities in health, beyond what individual risk factors alone would predict (Burris and Hacker 2017; Chae et al. 2018; Orchard and Price 2017). All of these factors capture elements of "institutional" or structural racism, and a number of articles have attempted to operationalize the concept and measure the effects on birth outcomes.[3]

In addition to the foci on racism at the individual and "structural" levels, a largely separate research stream has explored potential social policy and income-support mechanisms on the assumption that these might disrupt the pathway between lower socioeconomic status (SES) and health (Hoynes, Miller, and Simon 2015; Riley et al. 2021; Strully 2011). Studies of antipoverty polices such as Aid to Families with Dependent Children/Temporary Aid for Needy Families (AFDC/TANF) and Medicaid participation in the Special Supplemental Nutrition Program for Women, Infants, and Children (Kowaleski-Jones and Duncan 2002) have produced results that we might expect: social policies improve birth outcomes (Almond, Hoynes, and Schanzenbach 2011). A number of articles have found that the earned income tax credit (EITC) is associated with better health among infants (Hamad and Rehkopf 2015; Hoynes, Miller, and Simon 2015; Markowitz et al. 2017; Strully, Rehkoph, and Zuan 2011; Wagenaar et al. 2019) and that higher minimum wages are associated with better birth outcomes.

Our contribution builds on this extant multidisciplinary literature and on an insight drawn from lessons of African American political history. From the New Deal era to the present, a broad array of African American thinkers and activists who pushed for racial equality emphasized a multifaceted agenda: broad and equitable social welfare provision for all, full

2. See Mutambudzi, Meyer, Reisine, and Warren (2017).

3. See Chambers et al. (2019); Chambers et al. (2020); Krieger et al. (2020); Janevic et al. (2021).

employment, and antidiscrimination law and public policy. Mainstream civil rights organizations, labor unions, and more radical groups insisted that federal provision of social welfare and employment were *preconditions* to advancing racial equality. Indeed, the 1963 March on Washington was for "Jobs and Freedom" and called for full employment, a New Deal style of public works, higher minimum wages, and school desegregation, in addition to support for the Civil Rights Act (Hamilton and Hamilton 1997; Reed 2020a; Reed 2020b).

They did so with good reason. Federal power and authority matter more in terms of the social determinants of health in the United States and in addressing racial health disparities because macroeconomic policies, health care access, social policies of various kinds, workers' rights, the making and enforcement of antidiscrimination law, and tax policies that promote income (and wealth) redistribution are all most effectively accomplished as implementations of national policies. Indeed, when the federal government addressed racial and class inequalities in the 1960s through the War on Poverty and Great Society programs, and coupled those efforts with antidiscrimination law, health disparities narrowed, especially for Black women and infants (Almond, Chay, and Greenstone 2007; Hahn et al. 2018; Kaplan, Ranjit, and Burgard 2008; Krieger et al. 2013).

By 1980 and the election of Ronald Reagan as US president, the nation had moved away from 1960s-era social and economic policies and in the direction of neoliberal ones. This meant relatively flat minimum wages, less federal protection for civil rights and workers' rights, deregulation of markets, and trade deals that facilitated corporate mobility to lower-wage economies, all of which resulted in widening economic inequality and persistent racial disadvantage (Osterman 1999; Kalleberg 2011).[4]

During this time, states experimented with and sometimes extended a range of social welfare policies that impact health outcomes (Howard 2007)[5], but policy design and generosity have varied significantly across the 50 states (Howard 2007; Campbell 2014). Bruch, Meyers, and Gornick (2018) looked at 10 federal-state programs and found consistent cross-state inequalities in provision. They also found that, after the Personal Responsibility and Work Opportunity Reconciliation Act of 1996, the federal government's devolution of authority over the administration of these programs *increased inequalities in cross-state provision*. This meant less

4. On states, unionization, and poverty, see Brady, Bakers, and Finnigan (2013).

5. Parolin (2019) looked at data from 2012 to 2014 and found that differences in cash assistance from TANF, attributable to Black composition in a particular state, accounted for 15% of the Black-white child poverty gap.

direct cash assistance to the poor and the establishment of work requirements and punitive sanctions for not complying (Soss, Fording, and Schram 2011).[6]

We set out to examine the question of whether more generous social welfare provision among the 50 states might have an impact on Black and white low birth weight and preterm birth as well as the Black-white gap, particularly in the period following the Personal Responsibility and Work Opportunity Reconciliation Act of 1996. Given that birth outcomes follow a socioeconomic gradient, we also wondered whether the impact of social welfare policies differs by level of formal education for Black and white mothers.

Three articles have covered similar ground. Hoynes, Miller, and Simon (2015) used a difference-in-difference model to explore how the state expansion of the state EITC in 1993 impacted rates of low birth weight for white, Black, and Hispanic mothers with no more than a high school education. The expansion lowered rates of low birth weight for all mothers; however, the effects were strongest for Black mothers and weakest for white mothers. Wagenaar and colleagues (2019) categorized the EITC into four types based on the amount of the payment (low vs. high) and whether payments are refundable. They found that the strongest form of EITC (high levels with a refund) were associated with decreased rates of low birth weight and longer gestation periods for all mothers; but the effects were stronger for Black mothers than for white mothers. As with Hoynes, Miller, and Simon, their sample was women with no more than a high school diploma. Wehby, Dave, and Kaestner (2019) examined how the state minimum wage impacts birth weight and gestation for white and nonwhite mothers. They found that a minimum wage increase was associated with decreased rates of low birth weight for both white and nonwhite mothers, although the effects were stronger for nonwhite mothers. They also found that minimum wage increases were associated with lower rates of preterm birth for white mothers but not nonwhite mothers.

Our research differs from the previous studies in important ways. The first is conceptual. We understand the persistent racial gap in birth outcomes as the result of racism—interpersonal and structural—and we consider social welfare provision as a potential intervention. Second, we consider a broader set of policies that include safety net programs such as AFDC/TANF along with two that increase income through labor force

6. This is a period when the federal government's approach to providing housing to low-income Americans devolved in a way that gave states greater discretion over how public dollars were spent (Schwartz 2015).

participation—the minimum wage and the EITC, which we examine simultaneously.[7] Fourth, we operationalize the EITC in actual dollar amounts available to residents of specific states. Finally, and to weigh the impact of social policies *within* race, we stratify both the mother's race and her level of education.

Our study takes advantage of a dataset that allows us to include outcomes for every US live birth between 1994 and 2017—more than 60 million in total—along with detailed information about the mothers, including race/ethnicity, age, education level, prior pregnancies, prenatal care, and smoking behavior. We have data from the same period on state policies that aim to simultaneously mitigate economic inequality and assist low-income families with meeting basic economic needs. These include the EITC, the minimum wage, AFDC/TANF coverage, housing assistance, and Medicaid/Children's Health Insurance Program (CHIP). This interval of time captures significant changes in the US political economy in terms of tax policy, trade, workers' rights, minimum wages, and social welfare provision, and more specifically in the policies mentioned above. For instance, AFDC, one key element of the economic safety net, underwent dramatic revisions in 1996 with the introduction of the Personal Responsibility and Work Opportunities Reconciliation Act. The EITC expanded during this period.

Data and Sample

We use the National Vital Statistics System natality files from 1994 to 2017, compiled by the National Center for Health Statistics at the Centers for Disease Control and Prevention. These data, which are drawn from United States Standard Certificates of Live Birth, provide individual-level information on all infants born in the United States during this period. Demographic characteristics of the mother and infant as well as information on prenatal care and smoking during pregnancy are included in the dataset. We restrict the sample to singleton births to non-Hispanic white or non-Hispanic Black mothers. Mother's race is missing for less than 0.1% of the sample.[8] We include data from the 50 states but exclude Washington, DC.

7. Wehby, Dave, and Kaestner (2019) control for EITC but do not discuss the effects.

8. The variable for Hispanic/Latino ethnicity was missing for 0.75% of Black mothers and 1.22% of white mothers. For the analysis presented in the article, we exclude mothers for whom Hispanic/Latino ethnicity is missing. However, birth certificates where information on Hispanic ethnicity for the mother are missing may be much more likely to indicate non-Hispanic mothers. Therefore, we conducted a sensitivity analysis by estimating models where we include observations for Black and white mothers with missing data on Hispanic ethnicity. The results are extremely similar to those reported and are available on request.

We originally planned to use a sample consisting of all live births from 1980 to 2017, with state policy variables measured in each year from 1980 to 2017. However, because of the high correlation between the EITC and calendar year prior to 1994, we truncated our sample to produce reliable estimates for the EITC. It should be noted that when using the sample from 1980 to 2017, the findings for the other state policy variables were very similar to the results presented in this article.[9]

Our state-level policy information is drawn from several sources. We use information on EITC and minimum wage policies for 1994–2017 from the University of Kentucky Poverty Research Center's National Welfare Data set. We use data from the Annual Social and Economic Supplements to the Current Population Survey for 1992–2017 to create our additional state policy measures. Finally, we use data compiled by the US Department of Commerce and the US Census Bureau on state revenue and expenditures from 1994 to 2017.

Measures

Outcome Variables

We use two outcome variables: the first is a binary indicator of whether the infant was low birth weight (<2500 g) or not low birth weight (≥2500 g), and the second is a measure of whether the birth was preterm. We define preterm birth as gestation of fewer than 37 weeks.

Individual-Level Covariates

We measure the education of the mother as a series of five categories: did not complete elementary school, completed elementary school but did not graduate from high school, high school diploma, some college education, and bachelor's degree or more. We also include measures for the marital status of the mother (married vs. not married), the mother's age in years, whether this is the first live birth for that mother, and the sex of the infant. To allow for a nonlinear relationship between mother's age and our outcomes, we include both a linear and a squared term for the mother's age. In addition, we include a measure for the extent of prenatal care the mother received. Prenatal care is coded as adequate if this care began during the first two trimesters and inadequate otherwise. We also include a variable for whether the mother smoked during pregnancy. Finally, we include variables for the month and calendar year of the birth. To allow for flexibility in

9. Results are available on request.

changes over time, month and year are modeled as nominal categorical variables (e.g., month and year fixed effects).

State-Level Policy Variables

We include five state-level policy variables. All of these are time-varying (annual) measures for each year from 1994 to 2017 and are based on the state in which the mother resided at the time of the birth. Each of these policies is a key element of the social safety net designed to help low-income families meet basic economic needs.

- *Minimum wage*. This measure is the state minimum wage adjusted for annual inflation by the region-specific Consumer Price Index (CPI).
- *EITC*. This measure is the maximum level of earned income tax credit, including both the federal and the state-specific portions, that an individual with three dependents is eligible for in each state in each year. Our EITC measure is adjusted for annual inflation by the region-specific CPI provided by the Bureau of Labor Statistics. The base CPI year is 1983. The EITC is measured in $100s.
- *AFDC/TANF coverage*. This measure is a ratio. The numerator is the number of households in the state receiving AFDC/TANF, and the denominator is the number of households with children younger than the age of 18 in the state whose income falls below the federal poverty level.
- *Housing assistance*. This measure is a ratio. The numerator is the number of households in the state receiving a rent subsidy from the federal, state, or local government. The denominator is the number of households in the state with incomes below the federal poverty level.
- *Medicaid/CHIP*. This measure is a ratio. The numerator is the number of individuals in the state receiving Medicaid or CHIP. The denominator is the number of individuals in the state living in households with incomes below the federal poverty level.[10]

Additional State-Level Variables

To capture the general macroeconomic context, we include a measure of the state poverty rate and state unemployment rate in each year. We also

10. We considered using a sixth variable to measure the level of AFDC/TANF benefits provided by the state. Unfortunately, this variable produced high levels of multicollinearity, rendering the results unreliable. We were forced to drop it from the model.

include two variables to capture state levels of spending that benefit all individuals but are not specifically part of the social safety net: annual measures of state health/hospital expenditures and education expenditures. The education measure includes both K–12 and higher education spending. Health/hospital and education expenditures are measured in $1,000s per capita. We also include annual measures of the fraction of the population aged 18 years or younger and the fraction of the state population aged 65 or older. We include these variables as they may influence the level of spending on health and education. Finally, we include a time-invariant indicator (0/1) variable for each state (e.g., state-level fixed effects) that allows us to capture any time-invariant, unobserved, state-level characteristics that may influence gestation and birth weight.

Missing Data

For each model, we exclude cases with missing data on the outcome variable (low birth weight or preterm birth). We also restrict the analysis to cases with complete information on mother's race, age, education level, marital status, child's sex, and live birth order. Missing data on most of these characteristics is minimal. There is no missing data on mother's age or the sex of the infant. Marriage, live birth order, gestation, low birth weight, and preterm birth are missing for less than 1% of observations for both non-Hispanic Black and non-Hispanic white mothers. Education is missing for a slightly larger percentage of the sample: 3.1% of non-Hispanic Black mothers and 2.3% of non-Hispanic white mothers. Prenatal care received is missing for 4.5% of non-Hispanic Black mothers and 2.3% of non-Hispanic white mothers. We include cases with missing data on prenatal care along with an indicator variable for missing prenatal care information. Data on smoking during pregnancy is missing for 3.9% of non-Hispanic Black mothers and 5.6% of non-Hispanic white mothers. We include cases with missing data on smoking and also include an indicator of missing data on smoking in our models. In terms of the policy data, New Hampshire in 2011 and Rhode Island in 2015 are missing the AFDC/TANF coverage measure because of incomplete information on the number of households with children whose income is below the federal poverty level. Missouri in 1999 is missing data on housing assistance coverage because of incomplete information on rent subsidies. We exclude observations from the aforementioned states in the years in which they are missing policy data.

Analytic Strategy

We estimate logistic regression models for preterm birth and low birth weights separately for non-Hispanic Black and non-Hispanic white mothers. These models allow the impact of both state policy variables as well as individual covariates to vary by race. We then further stratify the models by education level, separately estimating models for mothers of each race who do not have a high school diploma, who have a high school diploma (no college education), who have some college education, and who have a bachelor's or graduate degree. To interpret the magnitude of the results, we use the coefficients from these models to microsimulate a series of predicted probabilities for each outcome, where we allow values for the five policy variables of interest to vary.[11] We estimate predicted probabilities at the 1st percentile, 50th percentile, and 99th percentile of the values on each policy variable. Percentiles are derived from our combined sample of non-Hispanic Black and non-Hispanic white mothers from 1994 to 2017. We use STATA version 16 for all analysis.

Results

Trends over Time in Low Birth Weight and Preterm Births by Race

Figures 2 and 3 show trends over time in rates of low birth weight and preterm birth respectively. There were only minor fluctuations in rates of low birth weight from 1994 to 2017, with no substantial trend over time. Low birth weight rates for non-Hispanic Black mothers were consistently more than twice the rates for non-Hispanic white mothers. The patterns for preterm birth are somewhat different. Between 1994 and 2017 the rates of preterm birth for non-Hispanic Black mothers dropped by about 2 percentage points (from 17.0% to 14.9%). The rates did rise slightly (from 14.4% to 14.9%) between 2015 and 2017; there is no way knowing if this trend will continue. For non-Hispanic white mothers, the rates of preterm birth rose and then fell during this time period; rates in 2017 were half a percentage point higher than in 1994 (8.5% vs. 8.0%). The gap between non-Hispanic Black mothers and non-Hispanic white mothers narrowed during this time period. Nevertheless, in 2017, rates for non-Hispanic Black mothers were still 1.75 times as high as those for non-Hispanic white mothers.

11. For these predicted probabilities, each observation retains its values on the other covariates. A predicated probability is calculated for each observation, and we then take the average of these individual predicted probabilities.

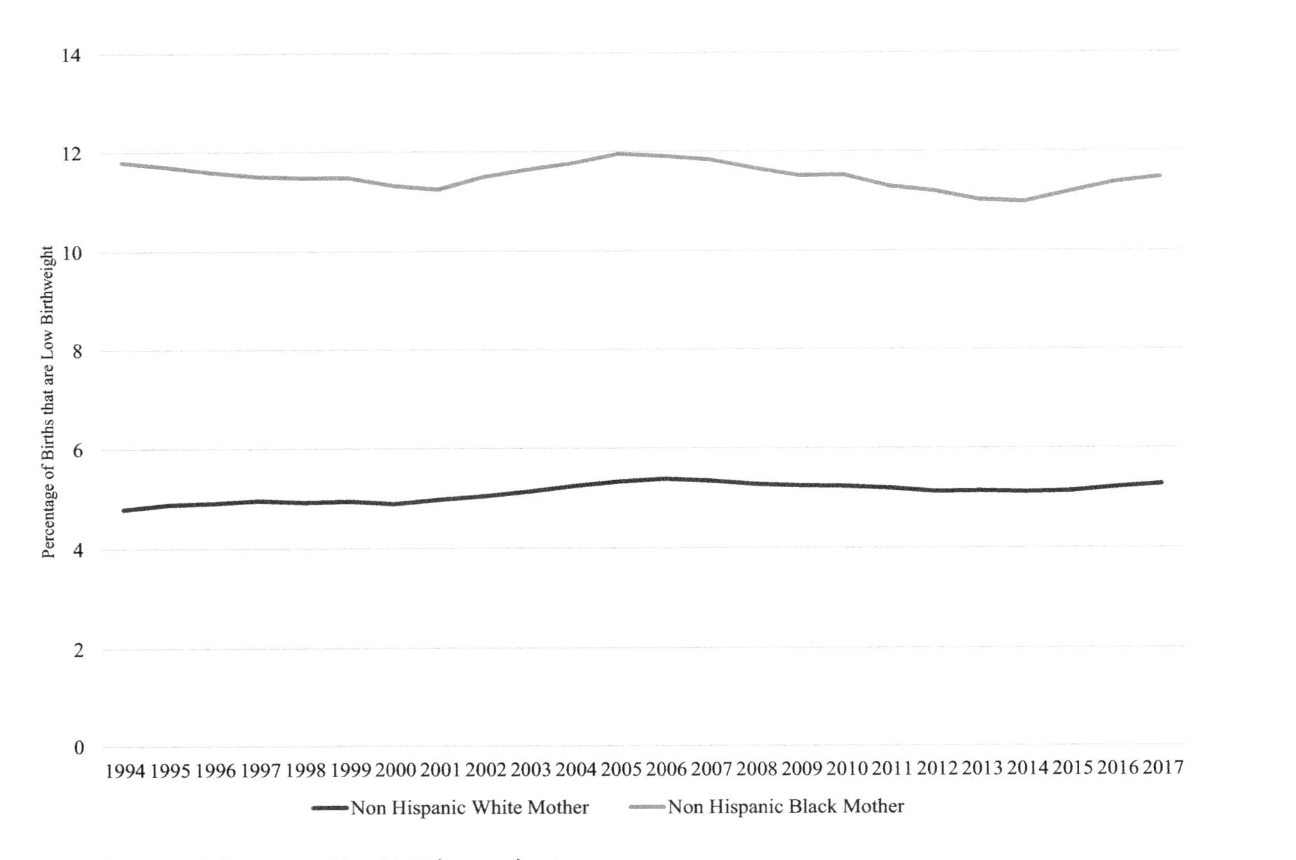

Figure 2 Low birth weight rates 1994–2017 by mother's race.

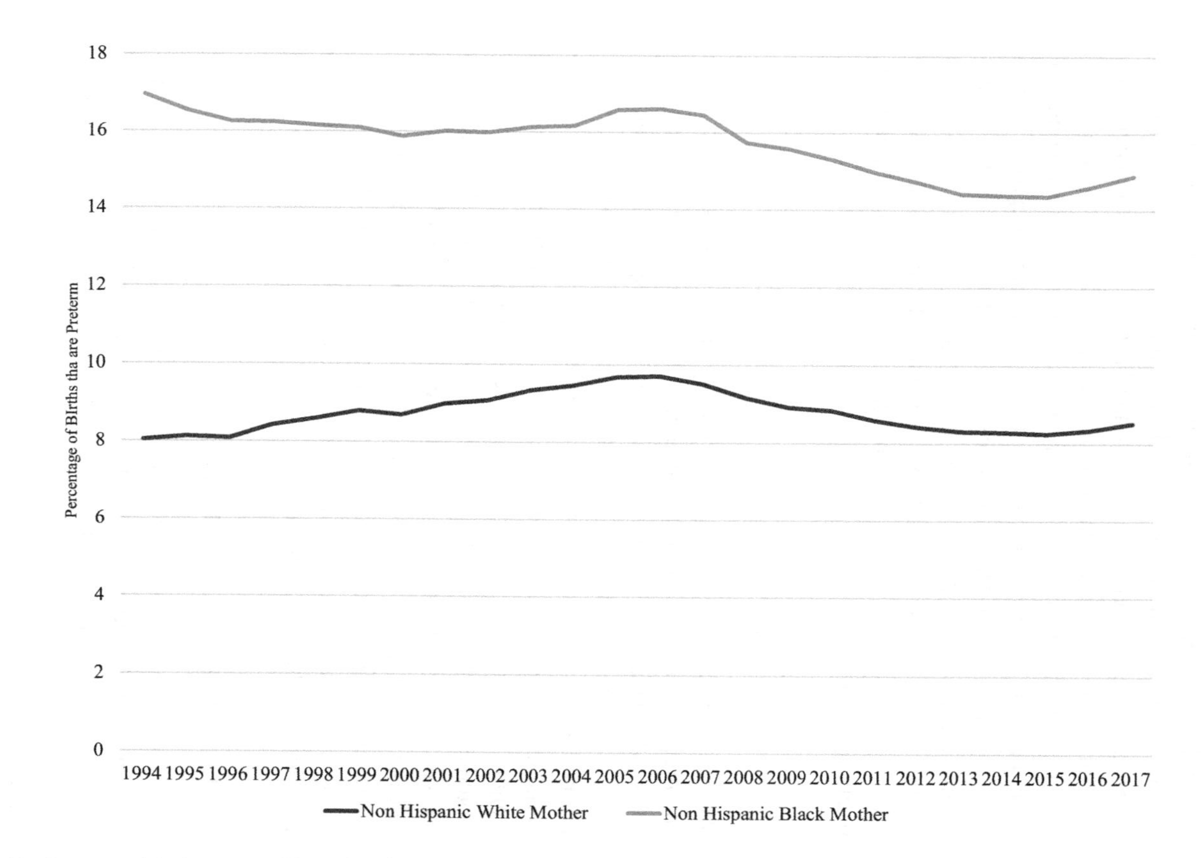

Figure 3 Preterm birth rates 1994–2017 by mother's race.

Descriptive Statistics

We see from table 1 that the rates of low birth weight and preterm birth are higher for non-Hispanic Black mothers than for non-Hispanic white mothers. Educational attainment and marriage rates are higher for non-Hispanic white mothers. Relative to non-Hispanic Black mothers, non-Hispanic white mothers are more than twice as likely to be married, are 11 percentage points more likely to have at least a high school diploma, and are more than twice as likely to have at least a bachelor's degree. The great majority of both non-Hispanic Black and non-Hispanic white mothers receive adequate prenatal care, although rates are twice as high for non-Hispanic white mothers. Finally, non-Hispanic Black mothers are about 3 years younger on average and are just over 5 percentage points less likely to smoke.

Bivariate Regression Models

We first estimate bivariate logistic regression models for low birth weight and preterm birth, each model containing one of our five key policy variables. Models are estimated separately for non-Hispanic Black and non-Hispanic white mothers. These results are presented in appendix table A1. For both outcomes and both samples of mothers, increases in each policy variable are associated with declines in both preterm birth and low birth weight. All results are statistically significant at $p < .001$, which is what we would expect. These models are a useful starting point, but they include no individual covariates or year or state fixed effects. Therefore, we cannot rule out the possibility that associations between policies and outcomes are the result of other state characteristics or characteristics of the individuals living within these states that are correlated with both the policies in question and the birth outcomes.

Multivariate Regression Models

We then estimate models including both non-Hispanic white and non-Hispanic Black mothers to show the overall racial disparities in low birth weight and preterm birth, net of any differences in demographic characteristics, prenatal care, and social welfare policies in the states in which these mothers live. As table 2 shows, the likelihoods of low birth weight and preterm birth are statistically significantly higher for non-Hispanic

Table 1 Mean (Standard Deviation) or Percentage, 1994–2017

	Non-Hispanic Black mothers (13,051,622)	Non-Hispanic white mothers (50,602,456)
Low birth weight	11.4%	5.1%
Preterm birth	15.7%	8.7%
Female infant	49.2%	48.7%
Mother's education:		
Elementary school	2.3%	1.6%
Some high school	20.1%	9.5%
High school diploma	36.4%	27.7%
Some college	27.3%	27.0%
Bachelor's degree	12.9%	34.2%
Married	29.6%	74.3%
Prenatal care:		
Prenatal care adequate	88.2%	94.8%
Prenatal care inadequate	7.7%	3.1%
Prenatal care missing	4.1%	2.1%
First live birth	39.0%	42.1%
Mother's age	25.7 (6.2)	28.2 (5.9)
Smoking during pregnancy:		
Mother smoked	7.8%	13.2%
Smoking missing	3.9%	5.6%
State variables:		
EITC ($100s)	25.27 (3.68)	25.11 (3.89)
AFDC/TANF coverage	0.91 (0.59)	0.98 (0.72)
Medicaid/CHIP coverage	1.00 (0.26)	1.03 (0.28)
Housing assistance coverage	0.11 (0.06)	0.12 (0.06)
Minimum wage ($s)	3.01 (0.41)	3.04 (0.43)
Poverty rate (measured as a fraction)	0.14 (0.03)	0.13 (0.03)
Unemployment rate	5.87 (1.86)	5.70 (1.85)
Education expenditures ($1000s per capita)	0.76 (0.16)	0.78 (0.17)
Health/hospital expenditures ($1000s per capita)	0.17 (0.06)	0.16 (0.06)
Fraction of population aged 65 and older	0.13 (0.02)	0.13 (0.02)
Fraction of population aged 18 and younger	0.27 (0.02)	0.27 (0.02)

Note: EITC = earned income tax credit; AFDC = Aid to Families with Dependent Children; TANF = Temporary Assistance for Needy Families; CHIP = Children's Health Insurance Program.

Black mothers as compared to non-Hispanic white mothers. The model-predicted probabilities of low birth weight are 10.3% for non-Hispanic Black mothers and 5.2% for non-Hispanic white mothers. The model-predicted probabilities of preterm birth are 14.0% for non-Hispanic Black mothers and 9.0% for non-Hispanic white mothers. These regression

Table 2 Low Birth Weight and Preterm Birth, 1994–2017

	Low birth weight		Preterm birth	
	Coeff	SE	Coeff	SE
Non-Hispanic Black mother	0.75058***	(0.00128)	0.49549***	(0.00107)
Female infant	0.18825***	(0.00104)	−0.10680***	(0.00084)
Elementary school	0.13750***	(0.00360)	0.07559***	(0.00302)
Some high school	0.17525***	(0.00161)	0.13486***	(0.00137)
Some college	−0.15478***	(0.00140)	−0.09266***	(0.00113)
Bachelor's degree	−0.42011***	(0.00169)	−0.30421***	(0.00132)
Married	−0.25061***	(0.00133)	−0.20976***	(0.00109)
First live birth	0.44025***	(0.00117)	0.08674***	(0.00095)
Mother's age	−0.01079***	(0.00068)	−0.04629***	(0.00056)
Mother's age squared	0.00071***	(0.00001)	0.00117***	(0.00001)
Inadequate prenatal care	0.29564***	(0.00216)	0.28106***	(0.00184)
Missing prenatal care	0.54437***	(0.00263)	0.39944***	(0.00233)
Smokes	0.65141***	(0.00144)	0.22448***	(0.00127)
Smoking missing	0.15911***	(0.00336)	0.09402***	(0.00270)
State variables:				
EITC	−0.00079	(0.00043)	−0.00253***	(0.00035)
AFDC/TANF coverage	0.00088	(0.00102)	−0.00153	(0.00083)
Medicaid/CHIP coverage	0.02312***	(0.00416)	0.02298***	(0.00336)
Housing assistance coverage	−0.00582	(0.01348)	−0.02428*	(0.01083)
Minimum wage	0.00052	(0.00217)	0.00427*	(0.00175)
Poverty rate	−0.00303***	(0.00045)	0.00190***	(0.00036)
Unemployment rate	−0.00163	(0.00084)	−0.00035	(0.00068)
Education expenditures	−0.00086	(0.01064)	−0.02548**	(0.00860)
Public health/hospital expenditures	0.02471	(0.01790)	−0.16414***	(0.01449)
Fraction of population aged 65 or over	0.26611***	(0.06862)	−0.17107**	(0.05524)
Fraction of population Aged 18 or younger	−0.10107	(0.06288)	−0.53424***	(0.05048)
Constant	−3.52303***	(0.02855)	−1.85009***	(0.02307)
Observations	63,637,177		63,446,968	

*** $p<0.001$, ** $p<0.01$, * $p<0.05$

Note: Models in table 2 include month, year, and state fixed effects. Reference categories: high school diploma, adequate prenatal care. EITC = earned income tax credit; AFDC = Aid to Families with Dependent Children; TANF = Temporary Assistance for Needy Families; CHIP = Children's Health Insurance Program.

models do not allow for the fact that the impact of the policy variables and individual covariates may vary by the mother's race. To incorporate this difference, we then estimate models separately for non-Hispanic Black and non-Hispanic white mothers.[12]

Table 3 shows the results for models of low birth weight and preterm birth, estimated separately for non-Hispanic Black and non-Hispanic white mothers. For both groups, the impact of individual covariates is in the expected directions. For both groups of mothers, low birth weight and preterm birth are more frequent for mothers at older ages. The risk of low-birth-weight births rises with age from age 11 for non-Hispanic Black mothers and from age 8 for non-Hispanic white mothers, effectively the earliest years for which pregnancy can occur. Preterm births rise with age from age 22 for non-Hispanic Black mothers and age 20 for non-Hispanic white mothers.[13] Risk of low birth weight and preterm birth are also higher for unmarried mothers, mothers who have less formal education, mothers who have received inadequate prenatal care, and mothers who smoke during pregnancy. Low birth weights are more frequent, although preterm births are less frequent for female infants.

The impacts of the state-level controls are less consistent. For instance, educational expenditures are associated with a decrease in low birth weight and preterm birth for non-Hispanic Black mothers, but not for non-Hispanic white mothers. Health expenditures are associated with lower rates of preterm birth for both samples of mothers and with low birth weight for non-Hispanic white mothers. Health expenditures are, however, associated with an increase in low birth weight for non-Hispanic Black mothers. It is important to note that this measure not only captures state investment in health care but also represents the number of sick people in the state who may need care. This may help to explain the positive association with low birth weight.

The results for our key state policy variables of interest are as follows. Increases in the level of the EITC and AFDC/TANF coverage are associated with a statistically significant lower risk of low birth weight and preterm birth for non-Hispanic Black mothers. For non-Hispanic white mothers, the EITC is associated with a statistically significant lower risk of preterm birth only. AFDC/TANF coverage is actually associated with

12. Another option is to include interaction terms between the mother's race and all other variables in the model. However, such models introduced very high levels of multicollinearity and thus were difficult to interpret.

13. These calculations use the formula -b/2a for the age of lowest risk, where b is the coefficient for the linear term and a is the coefficient for the squared term. This is the formula for the age of lowest risk when the squared term is positive and the linear term is negative.

Table 3 Non-Hispanic Black and Non-Hispanic White Mothers: Low Birth Weight and Preterm Birth, 1994–2017

	Low birth weight				Preterm birth			
	Non-Hispanic Black		Non-Hispanic white		Non-Hispanic Black		Non-Hispanic white	
	Coeff	SE	Coeff	SE	Coeff	SE	Coeff	SE
Female infant	0.22014***	(0.00176)	0.17081***	(0.00129)	–0.04018***	(0.00153)	–0.13538***	(0.00100)
Elementary school	0.03079***	(0.00597)	0.20834***	(0.00450)	0.12829***	(0.00506)	0.04548***	(0.00380)
Some high school	0.11576***	(0.00243)	0.22989***	(0.00215)	0.10880***	(0.00214)	0.14922***	(0.00179)
Some college	–0.10941***	(0.00230)	–0.17910***	(0.00177)	–0.09409***	(0.00201)	–0.09119***	(0.00137)
Bachelor's degree	–0.32309***	(0.00337)	–0.44564***	(0.00199)	–0.26500***	(0.00292)	–0.31064***	(0.00151)
Married	–0.24573***	(0.00232)	–0.23646***	(0.00163)	–0.20032***	(0.00200)	–0.20789***	(0.00130)
First live birth	0.32957***	(0.00205)	0.49531***	(0.00143)	–0.03433***	(0.00182)	0.13143***	(0.00111)
Mother's age	–0.02019***	(0.00113)	–0.01247***	(0.00087)	–0.07169***	(0.00099)	–0.04228***	(0.00070)
Mother's age squared	0.00088***	(0.00002)	0.00074***	(0.00001)	0.00166***	(0.00002)	0.00108***	(0.00001)
Inadequate prenatal care	0.24745***	(0.00307)	0.34111***	(0.00303)	0.26180***	(0.00270)	0.28828***	(0.00252)
Missing prenatal care	0.41357***	(0.00397)	0.65277***	(0.00349)	0.28616***	(0.00370)	0.47644***	(0.00300)
Smokes	0.56143***	(0.00289)	0.66594***	(0.00169)	0.22277***	(0.00274)	0.21757***	(0.00145)
Smoking missing	0.15702***	(0.00628)	0.16707***	(0.00401)	0.11603***	(0.00558)	0.10035***	(0.00311)
State variables:								
EITC	–0.00408***	(0.00074)	0.00095	(0.00052)	–0.00513***	(0.00066)	–0.00111**	(0.00041)
AFDC/TANF coverage	–0.00648**	(0.00200)	0.00321**	(0.00119)	–0.00547**	(0.00175)	0.00021	(0.00094)
Medicaid/CHIP coverage	0.00219	(0.00764)	0.02603***	(0.00498)	0.00594	(0.00671)	0.02066***	(0.00390)
Housing assistance coverage	0.05539*	(0.02445)	–0.01683	(0.01624)	0.06283**	(0.02138)	–0.02100	(0.01262)
Minimum wage	0.00103	(0.00378)	–0.00187	(0.00267)	0.01416***	(0.00332)	–0.00160	(0.00207)

Table 3 *(continued)*

	Low birth weight				Preterm birth			
	Non-Hispanic Black		Non-Hispanic white		Non-Hispanic Black		Non-Hispanic white	
	Coeff	SE	Coeff	SE	Coeff	SE	Coeff	SE
Poverty rate	−0.00053	(0.00076)	−0.00479***	(0.00056)	0.00321***	(0.00066)	0.00051	(0.00043)
Unemployment rate	−0.00353*	(0.00143)	0.00023	(0.00104)	0.00024	(0.00125)	−0.00041	(0.00081)
Education expenditures	−0.06311**	(0.01947)	0.02025	(0.01277)	−0.07671***	(0.01701)	−0.00008	(0.01003)
Public health/hospital expenditures	0.13947***	(0.03201)	−0.05534*	(0.02175)	−0.20286***	(0.02812)	−0.17051***	(0.01702)
Fraction of population aged 65 or over	0.13629	(0.12049)	0.26414**	(0.08393)	−0.14817	(0.10515)	−0.14959*	(0.06524)
Fraction of population aged 18 or younger	−0.24116*	(0.11110)	0.00483	(0.07673)	−0.67401***	(0.09658)	−0.31550***	(0.05959)
Constant	−2.42693***	(0.05015)	−3.60407***	(0.03503)	−0.86666***	(0.04381)	−2.00852***	(0.02741)
Observations	13,046,503		50,590,674		12,999,532		50,447,436	

*** $p < 0.001$, ** $p < 0.01$, * $p < 0.05$.

Note: Models include month, year, and state fixed effects. Reference categories: high school diploma, adequate prenatal care. EITC = earned income tax credit; AFDC = Aid to Families with Dependent Children; TANF = Temporary Assistance for Needy Families; CHIP = Children's Health Insurance Program.

Table 4 Values of Centiles for State Policy Variables, 1994–2017

	1st percentile	50th percentile	99th percentile
EITC ($100s)	16.90	23.93	37.03
AFDC/TANF coverage	0.12	0.89	3.61
Medicaid/CHIP coverage	0.59	0.98	1.99
Housing assistance coverage	0.02	0.10	0.31
Minimum wage ($s)	1.94	3.05	3.93

Note: 1st, 50th, and 99th percentiles for each policy variable are calculated with the entire sample of non-Hispanic Black and non-Hispanic white mothers. EITC = earned income tax credit; AFDC = Aid to Families with Dependent Children; TANF = Temporary Assistance for Needy Families; CHIP = Children's Health Insurance Program.

an increase in low birth weight rates for non-Hispanic white mothers; there is no association for preterm birth. The other three policy variables also have scattered statistically significant associations with birth outcomes that are in the opposite direction from what we would expect: Medicaid/CHIP coverage is associated with a higher rate of low birth weight and preterm birth for non-Hispanic white mothers. Housing assistance coverage is associated with a higher rate of low birth weight and preterm birth for non-Hispanic Black mothers. The minimum wage is associated with higher rate of preterm birth for non-Hispanic Black mothers.

Because of a sample size of more than 18 million non-Hispanic Black mothers and more than 70 million non-Hispanic white mothers, even trivial associations will be statistically significant. All results, especially those in unexpected directions, should be understood in this context.[14] We thus use predicted probabilities to examine the magnitude of these associations.

Table 4 shows the values for each state policy variable at the 1st, 50th, and 99th percentile. These percentiles are drawn from the entire sample of non-Hispanic Black and non-Hispanic white mothers from 1994 to 2017. We also calculated the percentiles using mothers of all race and ethnicities; the results were effectively identical. Table 5 shows the predicted probabilities of low birth weight and preterm births for non-Hispanic Black and non-Hispanic white mothers at the 1st, 50th, and 99th percentiles for each policy variable. All state policy variables are included for the sake of completeness; the statistical significance of the association between the

14. The bivariate correlations among all state-level variables are presented in appendix table A1. None of the correlations exceeds .51, with the exception of a fraction of the population aged 18 and under with a fraction of the population aged 65 and older. Those two variables can be considered analogous to two parameters for a categorical variable (e.g., age). They are correlated by definition. We also conducted tests of multicollinearity for the state policy variables. None exceeded a variance inflation factor of 10.

Table 5 Predicted Rates (%) of Low Birth Weight and Preterm Birth, 1994–2017

	1st percentile	50th percentile	99th percentile	Statistical significance
Non-Hispanic Black mothers: low birth weight				
EITC	11.8	11.5	10.9	($p<.001$)
AFDC/TANF coverage	11.5	11.4	11.2	($p<.01$)
Medicaid/CHIP coverage	11.4	11.4	11.4	(NS)
Housing assistance coverage	11.4	11.4	11.5	($p<.05$)
Minimum wage	11.4	11.4	11.4	(NS)
Non-Hispanic white mothers: low birth weight				
EITC	5.0	5.1	5.1	(NS)
AFDC/TANF coverage	5.1	5.1	5.1	($p<.01$)
Medicaid/CHIP coverage	5.1	5.1	5.2	($p<.001$)
Housing assistance coverage	5.1	5.1	5.1	(NS)
Minimum wage	5.1	5.1	5.1	(NS)
Non-Hispanic Black mothers: preterm birth				
EITC	16.2	15.7	14.9	($p<.001$)
AFDC/TANF coverage	15.7	15.7	15.5	($p<.01$)
Medicaid/CHIP coverage	15.6	15.7	15.7	(NS)
Housing assistance coverage	15.6	15.7	15.8	($p<.01$)
Minimum wage	15.5	15.7	15.8	($p<.001$)
Non-Hispanic white mothers: preterm birth				
EITC	8.8	8.8	8.6	($p<.01$)
AFDC/TANF coverage	8.7	8.7	8.7	(NS)
Medicaid/CHIP coverage	8.7	8.7	8.9	($p<.001$)
Housing assistance coverage	8.8	8.7	8.7	(NS)
Minimum wage	8.8	8.7	8.7	(NS)

Note: 1st, 50th, and 99th percentiles for each policy variable are calculated with the entire sample of non-Hispanic Black and non-Hispanic white mothers. Values in table 5 control for marital status, mother's age, education, prenatal care, mother's smoking, infant's gender, live birth order, month, year, and state fixed effects and all state-level variables. EITC = earned income tax credit; AFDC = Aid to Families with Dependent Children; TANF = Temporary Assistance for Needy Families; CHIP = Children's Health Insurance Program; NS = association is not statistically significant.

state policy variable and the birth outcome is shown in the right column of the table. As table 5 shows, other than for the EITC, the impact of the state policies on birth outcomes are generally very small.

For non-Hispanic Black mothers, the impact of the EITC on both low birth weight and preterm birth is substantial. As table 5 shows, at the 1st percentile of the EITC, the model-predicted low birth weight is 11.8%; this

Table 6 Predicted Rates of Low Birth Weight and Preterm Birth, 1994–2017

	Non-Hispanic Black mothers: low birth weight	Non-Hispanic white mothers: low birth weight	Non-Hispanic Black mothers: preterm birth	Non-Hispanic white mothers: preterm birth
Married	9.7	4.5	13.9	10.0
Not married	12.1	6.3	16.4	8.3
Elementary school	12.2	7.0	17.8	10.0
Some high school	13.1	7.2	17.6	11.0
High school diploma	11.8	5.8	16.0	9.6
Some college	10.7	4.9	14.8	8.8
Bachelor's degree	8.9	3.8	12.8	7.2
Aged 20 years	10.1	4.3	14.6	7.9
Aged 25 years	11.0	4.7	14.7	8.1
Aged 30 years	12.4	5.4	16.0	8.8
Aged 35 years	14.5	6.3	18.5	10.0
Prenatal care adequate	11.0	4.9	15.2	8.6
Prenatal care inadequate	13.6	6.8	18.9	11.1
Prenatal care missing	15.7	9.0	19.2	13.1
Smokes	14.8	8.3	15.7	10.3
Does not smoke	9.1	4.5	13.0	8.4
Smoking missing	10.5	5.2	14.4	9.2

Note: Values in table 6 control for marital status, mother's age, education, prenatal care, mother's smoking, infant's gender, live birth order, month, year, and state fixed effects and all state-level variables.

falls to 10.9% for the 99th percentile of the EITC. Preterm births are 16.2% at the 1st percentile of the EITC, dropping to 14.9% by the 99th percentile. As table 6 shows, these changes are approximately comparable to the impact of getting a high school diploma, obtaining some college education, and giving birth five years earlier in life.

For non-Hispanic Black mothers, none of the other state policy variables are associated with a change of more than 3 percentage points in predicted rates of low birth rate or preterm birth. Several of these associations are not statistically significant, as noted by (NS) on the table. For non-Hispanic white mothers, no state policy variable is associated with a change of more than 1 percentage point in low birth weight rates or a change of more than 2 percentage points in preterm birth rates. Most of these associations are not statistically significant.

Regression Models: Stratified by Education

To further disentangle the impact of public policies on racial and socioeconomic disparities in birth outcomes, we estimated models separately for non-Hispanic Black and non-Hispanic white mothers with less than a high school diploma, a high school diploma, some college, and a bachelor's degree or more. Model results are shown in appendix tables A3–A6. Results for the EITC are illustrated in Figure 4 (low birth weight) and figure 5 (preterm births).

Table A3 shows that for non-Hispanic Black mothers at all levels of education below the bachelor's degree, as the EITC increases there is a statistically significant decline in the likelihood of low birth weight. For non-Hispanic Black mothers with a bachelor's degree, there is no statistically significant association between the EITC and low birth weight. We see from figure 4 that the magnitude of this association is strongest among mothers with lower educational attainment. For non-Hispanic Black mothers without a high school diploma, model-predicted rates of low birth weight are 13.8% at the 1st percentile of EITC benefits; this falls to 12.6% when the mother lives in a state with EITC benefits at the 99th percentile. While non-Hispanic Black mothers with a high school diploma have lower rates of low birth weight overall, the magnitude of the association with the EITC is similar to that for mothers with no high school diploma. At the 1st percentile of the EITC, the predicted rate of low birth weight is 12.2%; this falls to 11.1% for the 99th percentile of the EITC. For non-Hispanic Black mothers with some college education, the corresponding drop is only 0.7 percentage points (from 10.9% to 10.2%). For non-Hispanic Black mothers with a bachelor's degree, the predicted rate of low birth rate is 8.9%, regardless of the value of the EITC.

The results are very different for non-Hispanic white mothers. As table A4 shows, for those who have at least a high school diploma, there is not a statistically significant relationship between the EITC and low birth rate. For non-Hispanic white mothers with no high school diploma, a more generous EITC benefit is associated with an increase in the rate of low birth weight and this relationship is statistically significant. As figure 4 shows, at the 1st percentile of the EITC, the predicted rate of low birth weight is 8.0%; this increases to 8.6% at the 99th percentile of the EITC.

Figure 4 also illustrates that non-Hispanic Black mothers with a bachelor's degree have higher model-predicted rates of low birth weight than non-Hispanic white mothers with no high school diploma. Even at the 99th percentile of the EITC, non-Hispanic Black mothers at any education level have higher rates of low birth weight than all non-Hispanic white mothers.

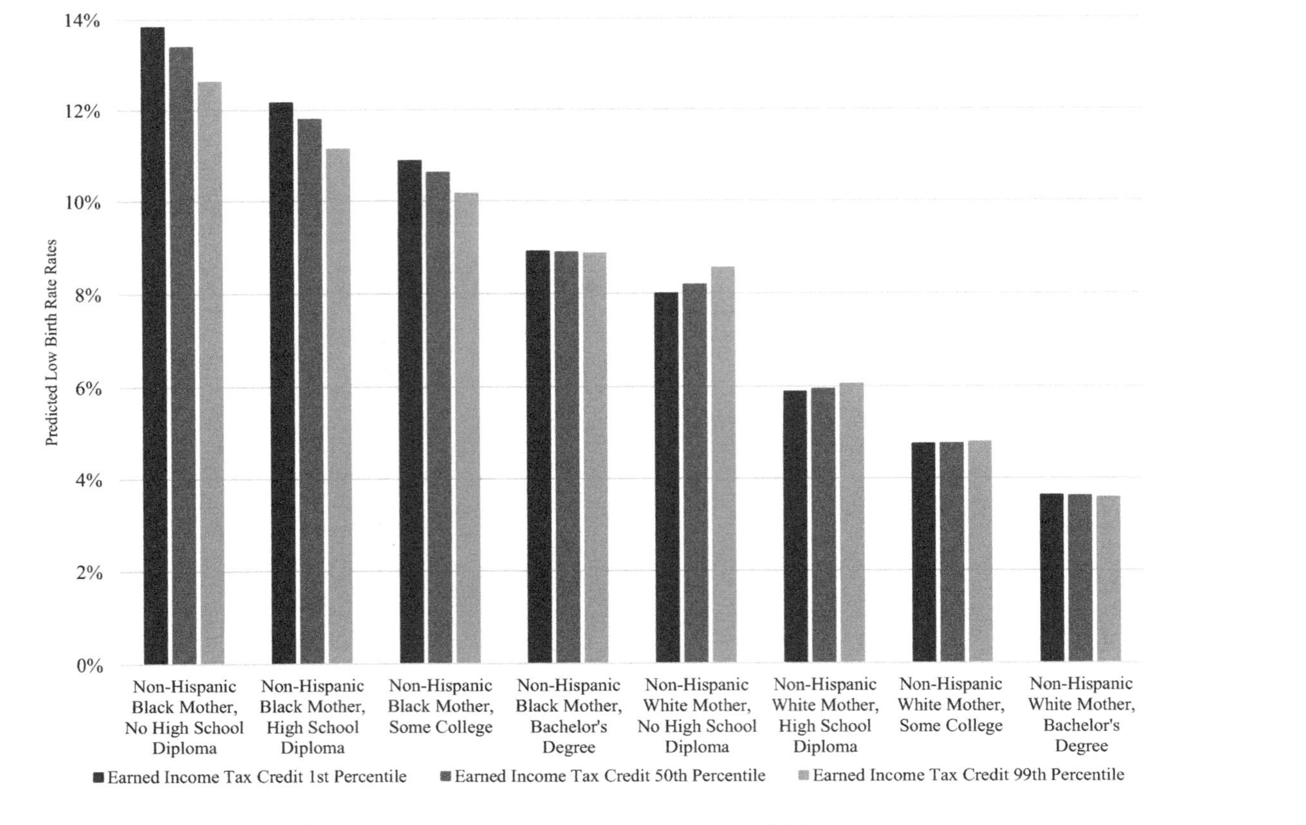

Figure 4 Predicted rates of low birth weight by race, education, and state EITC.

Note: 1st, 50th, and 99th percentiles for each policy variable are calculated with the entire sample of non-Hispanic Black and non-Hispanic white mothers. Rates in figure 4 control for marital status, mother's age, education, prenatal care, mother's smoking, infant's gender, live birth order, month, year, and state fixed effects and all state-level variables.

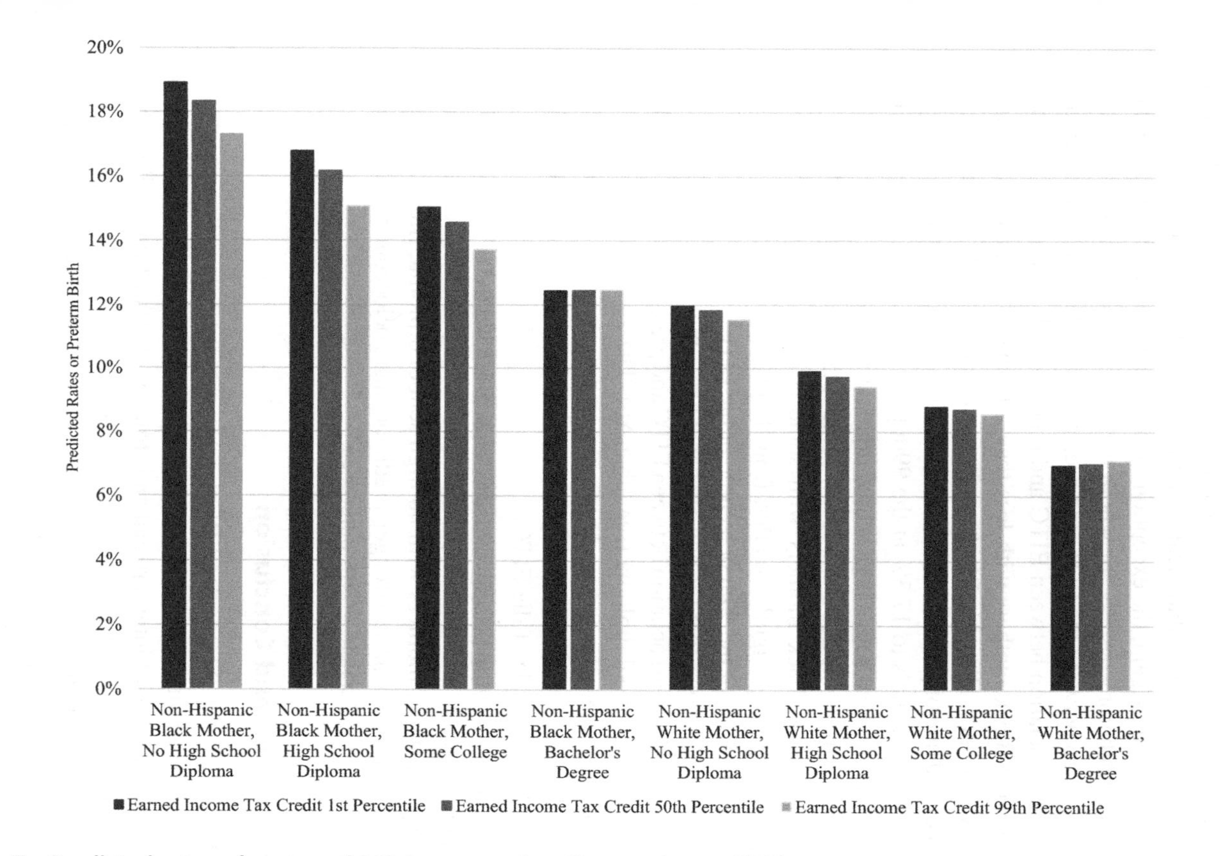

Figure 5 Predicted rates of preterm birth by race, education, and state EITC.

Note: 1st, 50th, and 99th percentiles for each policy variable are calculated with the entire sample of non-Hispanic Black and non-Hispanic white mothers. Rates in figure 5 control for marital status, mother's age, education, prenatal care, mother's smoking, infant's gender, live birth order, month, year, and state fixed effects and all state-level variables.

Results for preterm birth both mirror and diverge from those for low birth weight. Table A5 shows that for non-Hispanic Black mothers with all educational attainment levels below the bachelor's degree, as the EITC increases there is a statistically significant decline in the likelihood of preterm birth. Again, the exception to this is non-Hispanic Black mothers with a bachelor's degree, for whom there is not a statistically significant association between the EITC and preterm birth. However, the magnitude of the association between EITC and preterm birth is similar for all non-Hispanic Black mothers with less than a bachelor's degree. As figure 5 shows, for non-Hispanic Black mothers with no high school diploma, the predicted rate of preterm birth is 18.9% when at the 1st percentile of EITC benefits. This falls to 17.3% at the 99th percentile of EITC benefits. The trend for mothers with a high school diploma is very similar: 16.8% at the 1st percentile of the EITC and 15.1% at the 99th percentile of the EITC. For non-Hispanic Black mothers with some college education, the corresponding drop is slightly smaller: from 15.0% at the 1st percentile of the EITC to 13.7% at the 99th percentile of the EITC.

Table A5 shows that for non-Hispanic white mothers, the only statistically significant association between EITC and preterm birth is for mothers with a high school diploma (see table A6). The association between the EITC and preterm birth is modest for these mothers; at the 1st percentile of the EITC, the predicted rate of preterm birth is 10.0%; this falls to 9.4% at the 99th percentile of the EITC.

As with low birth weight, non-Hispanic Black mothers with a bachelor's degree have higher model-predicted rates of preterm birth than non-Hispanic white mothers with no high school diploma, illustrating that racial disparities are a stronger predictor than socioeconomic disparities in terms of influencing birth outcomes.

Discussion and Conclusion

We started with the puzzle of Black-white disparities in preterm birth and low birth weight and the understanding that SES did not adequately capture the gap because of interpersonal and structural (or "institutional") racism. We drew from civil rights history and captured a long-standing view that tackling racial injustice required federal and universal social welfare provision, full employment, and robust antidiscrimination law and policy. We then considered more than 60 million births over the course of three decades in relation to a specific set of federal policies that states administer and (sometimes) enhance.

Although our research uses a very robust data set, spanning 23 years of policy changes and including every US birth during that period, there are some limitations to this data. First, the individual-level data tell us whether mothers had access to prenatal health care but not whether they directly benefited financially from the particular policies we modeled. Thus, our results cannot say conclusively that *making use of* the financial resource of a particular policy benefits the birth outcomes for individual mothers. Rather, our research suggests that *having access to* the financial benefits of these policies is associated with improved birth outcomes. Relatedly, we do not have information on the household income level of the mothers; thus, we rely on education as a proxy for financial resources to stratify our model by socioeconomic class. While education is generally a good proxy for socioeconomic class, it does not completely capture diversity in financial resources.

Our results showed that the EITC reduces the risk of preterm birth and low birth weight for Black infants, and this association is strongest for Black mothers with the lowest levels of education. We found no association between the EITC and low birth weight for white infants, and the association between the EITC and preterm births for white infants was very small. Other safety net policies had minimal impact on birth outcomes for both Black and white infants.

It is not clear why the EITC has a stronger impact on birth outcomes relative to other social safety net policies, but it may be because the EITC has further reach than several other policies designed to assist low-income individuals and families. For instance, while only a limited number of housing assistance vouchers are available, there is no limit on the available coverage for the EITC; all employed individuals who earn below the specified threshold receive the credit. In addition, income eligibility restrictions for AFDC/TANF are much stricter than those for the EITC. For comparison, in 2017 22,220,000 individuals received the EITC (US Internal Revenue Service 2017), and monthly caseload averages for AFDC/TANF were 1,395,637 (US Department of Health and Human Services 2017). In 2016, 4.09 million households received governmental housing assistance from the Department of Housing and Urban Development (Kingsley 2017). In 2017, approximately 75 million people received health insurance through Medicaid (Rudowitz, Garfield and Hinton 2019). These numbers are not strictly comparable, as they operate on different scales. The EITC, AFDC/TANF, and housing assistance measures are *household-level* measures, as in general the eligibility rules are structured so one adult in each household can receive each of the aforementioned benefits. Medicaid is an individual-level benefit and applies to children as well as adults. We did supplemental calculations using Current Population Survey data from 2017 and found that 34,187,610 individuals older than the age of 18 received Medicaid. This is still by far the policy that benefits the greatest number of people. The EITC, however, has significantly greater reach than either AFDC/TANF or housing assistance.[15]

Our results confirm and buttress some prior findings as well as the historical, multipronged approach to addressing racial disadvantage that civil rights, labor leaders, and other (sometimes radical) activists pushed over the course of the 20th century. We found that supplementing the income of Black mothers through EITC at least modestly addresses racial and socioeconomic disparities in birth outcomes, especially for Black women who face the most disadvantage.

These results might be important for other reasons. They hold over a period that corresponds to the end of the "liberal consensus" and corresponding changes in social and economic policy that began with the Reagan Revolution. In a period of less market regulation, less progressive taxation, erosion of workers' rights, flatter wages, and a dramatic devolution of safety net policy after 1996, our findings are consistent: more generous EITC is modestly associated with adverse birth outcomes for Black infants.

The results matter because states vary in their levels and approaches to social welfare provision, and scholars have explored potential reasons for and consequences of those differences (Franko and Witko 2017; Hertel-Fernandez 2019; Yu, Jennings, and Butler 2019). We know that states with larger Black populations make less "welfare effort" and that higher Black caseloads mean more exclusionary, punitive welfare policies and less cash assistance (Matsubayashi and Rocha 2011; Parolin 2019; Soss, Fording, and Schram 2011). We share Mettler's concern about how "submerged"[16] social welfare policy (e.g., tax credits instead of direct subsidy) erodes the public's support for and understanding of governmental intervention, but in the case of the EITC that might be a virtue—it is less likely to be "racialized" than other safety net policies.

15. Since the AFDC/TANF data are monthly caseload averages, it is possible these numbers underestimate the total number of families who receive AFDC/TANF at some point in the year. However, we conducted supplemental analysis using the Current Population Survey, which asks individuals to report any income from AFDC/TANF in the prior year, and the numbers were very similar to those reported by the Department of Health and Human Services.

16. "Submerged" policies are "those that are located in the tax code or channeled through nongovernmental organizations, making government's role in providing them less obvious" (Mettler 2020).

At first glance, our results might be surprising because the EITC is targeted, but not to the population that faces the greatest inequality in birth outcomes. Long-standing and persistent racial gaps in birth outcomes could suggest that *only* specifically targeted interventions would change the outcome. But again, the theory and historical perspective that informed our analysis would predict some protective effect, albeit a smaller effect than would result from a more robust and generous social welfare provision.

Our results were surprising with respect to white infant outcomes. The EITC does not have the same consistent associations. Why would that be? Following Williams, we speculate that the variables we use to assess SES among Black and white mothers are not necessarily commensurate (Williams 2012). A variable like "formal education" does not capture everything relevant about the lived experience, past or present, of Black and white mothers of similar SES. It does not capture wealth differences or residential patterns that might result in more toxic exposures—all of which fall under the category of structural racism. Furthermore, as a result of the cumulative and co-occurring effects of racial, class, and gendered inequality, Black mothers experience greater cumulative "wear and tear" than their white counterparts, which Arline Gernonimus calls "weathering" (Geronimus et al. 2006). That Black women start from an initially more significant economic disadvantage tied to intergenerational processes might explain why the EITC has a consistently positive impact on Black infants, but less so for whites. Part of the stronger association between the EITC and birth outcomes for Black mothers is likely also because Black mothers are starting from such an extreme disadvantage relative to white mothers vis-à-vis birth outcomes. The EITC helps to mitigate this disparity.

The corollary is that social welfare policies and spending would likely need to be significantly more generous and robust to more dramatically affect both Black *and* white infant outcomes, and to attenuate racial differences in birth outcomes. As of this writing, the American Rescue Plan Act is a historic policy intervention regarding safety net and income support to families and might therefore serve as a natural experiment for future investigation. Our findings, and prior research, suggest that these developments will be beneficial for infant outcomes in general and are likely to attenuate the Black-white gap in health outcomes.

Additional research might also explore why none of the other policy variables showed a consistent significant association with birth outcomes and also why the EITC had limited impact on birth outcomes for white mothers. Because of the complexity of these issues, qualitative research could include interviews of Black and white mothers of various income levels about their pregnancy and prior lived experiences that might be relevant to birth outcomes. Mothers could be selected from states with generous social policies and states with more restrictive social policies. This research could explore the extent to which mothers made use of the public policies analyzed in this article, the trade-offs they make that may impact infant health (e.g., their nutritional status while they are pregnant, the number of prenatal care visits they receive, etc.) and the ways responses differ between Black and white mothers.

Despite the remaining research questions, the findings are still clear with respect to potential interventions. Higher EITC provision is consistently good for Black mothers and their infants, particularly those who are most disadvantaged.

■ ■ ■

Jessica Pearlman is director of research methods programs at the Institute for Social Science Research, University of Massachusetts Amherst. Her research focuses on racial, gender, and class inequalities in health outcomes; the labor market; and the criminal justice system. She also explores policy interventions designed to address these disparities.
jpearlman@issr.umass.edu

Dean E. Robinson is an associate professor of political science at the University of Massachusetts Amherst. He has published on Black politics and social thought as well as racial and class sources of health inequalities in the United States.
deanr@umass.edu

Acknowledgments

We thank three anonymous reviewers for their feedback. The authors contributed equally to the manuscript and are listed in alphabetical order.

References

Alhusen, Jeanne L., Kelly M. Bower, Elizabeth Epstein, and Phyllis Sharps. 2016. "Racial Discrimination and Adverse Birth Outcomes: An Integrative Review." *Journal of Midwifery and Women's Health* 61, no. 6: 707–20.

Almond, Douglas Vincent, Kenneth Y. Chay, and Michael Greenstone. 2007. "Civil Rights, the War on Poverty, and Black-White Convergence in Infant Mortality in the Rural South and Mississippi." MIT Department of Economics, Working Paper No. 07–04, February 7. dx.doi.org/10.2139/ssrn.961021.

Almond, Douglas, Hilary W. Hoynes, and Diane Whitmore Schanzenbach. 2011. "Inside the War on Poverty: The Impact of Food Stamps on Birth Outcomes." *Review of Economics and Statistics* 93, no. 2: 387–403.

Blumenshine, Philip, Susan Egerter, Colleen J. Barclay, Catherine Cubbin, and Paula A. Braveman. 2010. "Socioeconomic Disparities in Adverse Birth Outcomes: A Systematic Review." *American Journal of Preventive Medicine* 39, no. 3: 263–72.

Brady, David, Regina S. Bakers, and Ryan Finnigan. 2013. "When Unionization Disappears: State-Level Unionization and Working Poverty in the United States." *American Sociological Review* 78, no 5: 872–96.

Bruch, Sarah, Marcia Meyers, and Janet Gornick, 2018. "The Consequences of Decentralization: Inequality in Safety Net Provision in the Post-Welfare Reform Era." *Social Service Review* 92, no. 1: 3–35.

Burris, Heather H., and Michele R. Hacker. 2017. "Birth Outcome Racial Disparities: A Result of Intersecting Social and Environmental Factors." *Seminars in Perinatology* 41, no 5: 360–66.

Campbell, Andrea. 2014. *Trapped in America's Safety Net: One Family's Struggle.* Chicago: University of Chicago Press.

Carmichael, Stokely, and Charles Hamilton. 1967. *Black Power: The Politics of Liberation in America.* New York: Vintage Books.

Chae, David H., Sean Clouston, Conor D. Martz, Mark L. Hatzenbuehler, Hannah L. F. Cooper, Rodman Turpin, Seth Stephens-Davidowitz, and Michael R. Kramer. 2018. "Area Racism and Birth Outcomes among Blacks in the United States." *Social Science and Medicine* 199: 49–55.

Chambers, Brittany, Silvia E. Arabia, Helen Arega, Molly Altman, Rachel Berkowitz, Sky Feuer, Linda S. Franck, et al. 2020. "Exposures to Structural Racism and Racial Discrimination among Pregnant and Early Post-Partum Black Women Living in Oakland, California." *Stress and Health* 36, no. 2: 213–19.

Chambers, Brittany, Rebecca Baer, Monica McLemore, and Laura Jelliffe-Pawlowski. 2019. "Using Index of Concentration at the Extremes as Indicators of Structural Racism to Evaluate the Association with Preterm Birth and Infant Mortality—California, 2011–2012." *Journal of Urban Health* 96, no. 2: 159–70.

Collins, James W., Richard J. David, Rebecca Symons, Adren Handler, Stephen N. Wall, and Lisa Dwyer. 2000. "Low-Income African-American Mothers' Perception of Exposure to Racial Discrimination and Infant Birth Weight." *Epidemiology* 11, no. 3: 337–39.

David, Richard, and James Collins Jr. 1997. "Differing Birth Weight among Infants of US-Born Blacks, African-Born Blacks, and US-Born Whites." *New England Journal of Medicine* 337, no. 17: 1209–14.

David, Richard, and James Collins Jr. 2007. "Disparities in Infant Mortality: What's Genetics Got to Do with It?" *American Journal of Public Health* 97, no. 7: 1191–97.

Fields, Barbara J. 1990. "Slavery, Race, and Ideology in the United States of America." *New Left Review*, no. 181: 95–118. Franko, William, and Christopher Witko. 2017.

The New Economic Populism: How States Respond to Economic Inequality. New York: Oxford University Press.

Geronimus, Arline T., Margaret Hicken, Danya Keene, and John Bound. 2006. "'Weathering' and Age Patterns of Allostatic Load Scores among Blacks and Whites in the United States." *American Journal of Public Health* 96, no. 5: 826–33.

Hamad, Rita, and David Rehkopf. 2015. Poverty, Pregnancy, and Birth Outcomes: A Study of the Earned Income Tax Credit." *Paediatric and Perinatal Epidemiology* 29, no. 5: 444–52.

Hamilton, Dona Cooper, and Charles Hamilton. 1997. "Coping with the New Deal". In *The African-American Struggle for Civil and Economic Equality,* edited by Dona Cooper Hamilton and Charles Hamilton, 8–42. New York: Columbia University Press.

Hahn, Robert A., Benedict I. Truman, and D. R. Williams. 2018. "Civil Rights as Determinants of Public Health and Racial and Ethnic Health Equity: Health Care, Education, Employment, and Housing in the United States." *Social Science and Medicine—Population Health* 4: 17–24.

Hertel-Fernandez, Alex. 2019. *State Capture: How Conservative Activists, Big Businesses, and Wealthy Donors Reshaped the American States—And the Nation.* New York: Oxford University Press.

Howard, Christopher. 2007. *The Welfare State Nobody Knows: Debunking Myths About US Social Policy*. Princeton, NJ: Princeton University Press.

Hoynes, Hilary, Doug Miller, and David Simon. 2015. "Income, the Earned Income Tax Credit, and Infant Health." *American Economic Journal: Economic Policy* 7 , no. 1: 172–211.

Janevic, Teresa, Jennifer Zeitlin, Natalia N. Egorova, Paul Hebert, Amy Balbierz, Ann Marie Stroustrup, and Elizabeth A. Howell. 2021. "Racial and Economic Neighborhood Segregation, Site of Delivery, and Very Preterm Neonatal Morbidity and Mortality." *Journal of Pediatrics* 235: 116–23.

Kalleberg, Arne L. 2011. *Good Jobs, Bad Jobs: The Rise of Polarized and Precarious Employment Systems in the United States: 1970s–2000s*. New York: Russell Sage Foundation.

Kaplan, George A., Nalini Ranjit, and Sarah Burgard. 2008. "Lifting Gates, Lengthening Lives: Did Civil Rights Policies Improve the Health of African-American Women in the 1960s and 1970s?" In *Making Americans Healthier: Social and Economic Policy as Health Policy*, edited by Robert F. Schoeni, James S. House, George A. Kaplan, and Harold Pollack, 145–70. New York: Russell Sage Foundation.

Kawachi, Ichiro, Norman Daniels, and Dean E. Robinson. 2005. "Health Disparities by Race and Class: Why Both Matter." *Health Affairs* 24, no. 2: 343–52.

Kingsley, G. Thomas. 2017. "Trends in Housing Problems and Federal Housing Assistance." Urban Institute, October. www.urban.org/sites/default/files/publication/94146/trends-in-housing-problems-and-federal-housing-assistance.pdf.

Kowaleski-Jones, Lori, and Greg J. Duncan. 2002. "Effects of Participation in the WIC Program on Birthweight: Evidence from the National Longitudinal Survey of Youth." *American Journal of Public Health* 92, no. 5: 799–804.

Krieger, Nancy, Jarvis T. Chen, Brent Coull, Pamela D. Waterman, and Jason Beckfield. 2013. "The Unique Impact of Abolition of Jim Crow Laws on Reducing

Inequities in Infant Death Rates and Implications for Choice of Comparison Groups in Analyzing Societal Determinants of Health." *American Journal of Public Health* 103, no. 12: 2234–44.

Krieger, Nancy, Gretchen Van Wye, Mary Huynh, Pamela D. Wasserman, Gil Maduro, Wenhui Li, R. Charon Gwynn, Oxiris Brbot, and Mary T. Bassett. 2020. "Structural Racism, Historical Redlining, and Risk of Preterm Birth in New York City, 2013–2017." *American Journal of Public Health* 110, no. 7: 1046–53.

Markowitz, Sara, Kelli A. Komro, Melvin D. Livingston, Otto Lenhart, and Alexander C. Wagenaar. 2017. "Effects of State-Level Earned Income Tax Credit Laws in the US on Maternal Health Behaviors and Infant Health Outcomes." *Social Science and Medicine* 194: 67–75.

Matsubayashi, Tetsuya, and Rene R. Rocha. 2011. "Racial Diversity and Public Policy in the States." *Political Research Quarterly* 65, no 3: 600–14.

McGrady, Gene, John Sung, Diane Rowley, and Carol Hogue. 1992. "Preterm Delivery and Low Birth Weight among First-Born Infants of Black and White College Graduates." *American Journal of Epidemiology* 136, no. 3: 266–76.

Mettler, Suzanne, and Robert C. Lieberman. 2020. *Four Threats: The Recurring Crises of American Democracy*. New York: St. Martin's Press.

Mutambudzi, Miriam, John D. Meyer, Susan Reisine, and Nicholas Warren. 2017. "A Review of Recent Literature on Materialist and Psychosocial Models for Racial and Ethnic Disparities in Birth Outcomes in the US, 2000–2014." *Ethnicity and Health* 22, no. 3: 311–32.

Orchard, Jacob, and Joseph Price. 2017. "County-Level Racial Prejudice and the Black-White Gap in Infant Health Outcomes." *Social Science and Medicine* 181: 191–98.

Osterman, Paul. 1999. *The Changing Structure of the American Labor Market in Security Prosperity*. Princeton, NJ: Princeton University Press.

Parolin, Zachary. 2019. "Temporary Assistance for Needy Families and the Black-White Child Poverty Gap in the United States." *Socio-Economic Review* 19, no. 3: 1005–35.

Reed, Adolph Jr. 2020a. "Socialism and the Argument against Race Reductionism." *New Labor Forum* 29, no. 2: 36–43.

Reed, Toure. 2020b. "Toward Freedom: *The Case Against Race Reductionism.*" London: Verso.

Riley, Alicia R., Daniel Collin, Jacob M. Grambach, Jacqueline M. Torres, and Rita Hamad. 2021. "Association of US State Policy Orientation with Adverse Birth Outcomes: A Longitudinal Analysis." *Journal of Epidemiology and Community Health* 75, no. 7: 689–94.

Rosenthal, Lisa, and Marci Lobel. 2011. "Explaining Racial Disparities in Adverse Birth Outcomes: Unique Sources of Stress for Black American Women." *Social Science and Medicine* 72, no. 6: 977–83.

Rudowitz, Robin, Rachel Garfield, and Elizabeth Hinton. 2019. *10 Things to Know about Medicaid: Setting the Facts Straight*. Kaiser Family Foundation, March 6. www.kff.org/medicaid/issue-brief/10-things-to-know-about-medicaid-setting-the-facts-straight/.

Schwartz, Alex F. 2015. *Housing Policy in the United States*. 3rd ed. New York: Routledge.

Smedley, Brian. 2012. "The Lived Experience of Race and Its Health Consequences." *American Journal of Public Health* 102, no. 5: 933–35.

Soss, Joe, Richard Fording, and Sanford F. Schram. 2011. *Disciplining the Poor: Neoliberal Paternalism and the Persistent Power of Race*. Chicago: University of Chicago Press.

Strully, Kate W., David H. Rehkopf, and Ziming Zuan. 2011. "Effects of Prenatal Poverty on Infant Health: State Earned Income Tax Credits and Birth Weight." *American Sociological Review* 75, no. 4: 534–62.

US Department of Health and Human Services. 2017. "TANF Caseload Data 2017." September 26. www.acf.hhs.gov/ofa/data/tanf-caseload-data-2017.

US Internal Revenue Service. 2017. "Statistics for 2017 Tax Returns with EITC". www.eitc.irs.gov/eitc-central/statistics-for-tax-returns-with-eitc/statistics-for-2017-tax-returns-with-eitc (accessed November 17, 2021).

Wagenaar, Alexander C., Melvin D. Livingston, Sara Markowitz, and Kelli A. Komro. 2019. "Effects of Changes in Earned Income Tax Credit: Time-Series Analyses of Washington DC." *SSM—Population Health*, April. doi.org/10.1016/j.ssmph.2019.100356.

Wehby, George L., Dhaval M. Dave, and Robert Kaestner. 2019. "Effects of the Minimum Wage on Infant Health." *Journal of Policy Analysis and Management* 39, no. 2: 411–43.

Whitehead, Margaret. 1992. "The Concepts and Principles of Equity and Health." *International Journal of Health Services* 22, no. 3: 429–45.

Williams, David R. 2012. "Miles to Go before We Sleep: Racial Inequities in Health." *Journal of Health and Social Behavior* 53, no. 3: 279–95.

Yu, Jinhai, Edward T. Jennings Jr., and J. S. Butler. 2019. "Dividing the Pie: Parties, Institutional Limits, and State Budget Trade-Offs." *State Politics and Policy Quarterly* 19, no. 2: 236–58.

Mexican-Origin Women's Construction and Navigation of Racialized Identities: Implications for Health Amid Restrictive Immigrant Policies

Alana M. W. LeBrón
University of California, Irvine

Amy J. Schulz
University of Michigan

Cindy Gamboa
Angela Reyes
Detroit Hispanic Development Corporation

Edna Viruell-Fuentes
University of Illinois Urbana-Champaign

Barbara A. Israel
University of Michigan

Abstract This study examines how Mexican-origin women construct and navigate racialized identities in a postindustrial northern border community during a period of prolonged restrictive immigration and immigrant policies, and it considers mechanisms by which responses to racialization may shape health. This grounded theory analysis involves interviews with 48 Mexican-origin women in Detroit, Michigan, who identified as being in the first, 1.5, or second immigrant generation. In response to institutions and institutional agents using racializing markers to assess their legal status and policing access to health-promoting resources, women engaged in a range of strategies to resist being constructed as an "other." Women used the same racializing markers or symbols of (il)legality that had been used against them as a malleable set of resources to resist processes of racialization and to form, preserve, and affirm their identities. These responses include constructing an authorized immigrant identity, engaging in immigration advocacy, and resisting stigmatizing labels. These strategies may have different implications for health over time. Findings indicate the importance of addressing policies that promulgate or exacerbate racialization of Mexican-origin communities and other communities who experience growth through migration. Such policies include creating pathways to legalization and access to resources that have been invoked in racialization processes, such as state-issued driver's licenses.

Keywords immigration enforcement, immigrant policies, racialization, racism, health

Journal of Health Politics, Policy and Law, Vol. 47, No. 2, April 2022
DOI 10.1215/03616878-9518665

Understanding and addressing structural racism is central to reducing health inequities (Ford et al. 2019). Racialization is the active and dynamic process by which systems, institutions, and agents create and maintain subordinate and dominant racial groups, assign differential value to racial groups, and leverage symbols of divergent value to justify inequitable rights, opportunities, access to resources, and treatment (Omi and Winant 2015; Schwalbe et al. 2000). Racialization processes, including the conceptualization and categorization of race and the creation of policies and practices grounded in racialization, vary over time and place and have enduring impacts (Omi and Winant 2015). Historical and contemporary racialization processes have unique implications for how Latina/o subgroups identify, are defined, and negotiate systems of classification; ultimately, they have implications for health (LeBrón and Viruell-Fuentes 2020). In this article, we examine Mexican-origin women's construction, negotiation, and management of racialized and gendered identities within the context of a complex and interconnected web of restrictive immigration and immigrant policies in a northern border US community. We leverage these findings to more fully understand the public health literature regarding racialization, immigration and immigrant policies, and health.

Immigration and Immigrant Policies

US immigration policies, which shape opportunities to lawfully migrate to and remain in the United States, and immigrant policies, which are designed to influence the lives of US immigrants and immigrant communities, are manifestations of historical and contemporary racism and xenophobia (LeBrón and Viruell-Fuentes 2020; Wallace and De Trinidad Young 2018). For example, the Immigration Act of 1924 formalized the social construct of "illegal alien," established numerical quotas for immigration, and augmented attention to the national border and interior regions as spaces of social control of immigrants (Ngai 2004). Together, these events contributed to the extension of border enforcement efforts and large-scale deportations (Ngai 2004). A focus on controlling the southern US border and administrative discretion to prevent deportation of socially desirable immigrants contribute to the enduring construction of Mexican-origin peoples as unauthorized foreigners (Chavez 2013; Ngai 2004). Restrictive immigration policy in the 21st century includes the proliferation of border enforcement apparatuses, mass hyperpolicing and detention of immigrants, and collaborations between local law enforcement and federal immigration enforcement agencies to police immigrant communities in the interior of the United States (e.g., roadways, public transportation, occupational settings) (Coleman and Stuesse 2014; De Genova 2007; Miller 2014).

Restrictive immigrant policies are those that limit immigrants' rights, protections, opportunities, and access to resources on the basis of legal status (Wallace et al. 2019). The intersection of federal, state, and local immigrant policies shapes contexts of reception or exclusion for immigrants and immigrant communities (Wallace et al. 2019). A distinguishing feature of 21st-century immigrant policies is the infusion of immigrant policies into sectors that were previously relatively siloed from immigrant policies: health care, education, law enforcement, employment, and social welfare (Cruz Nichols, LeBrón, and Pedraza 2017; Pedraza, Cruz Nichols, and LeBrón 2017; Wallace and De Trinidad Young 2018). The extension of immigrant policies into these sectors is facilitated through technological advances that enable information sharing across agencies (Cruz Nichols, LeBrón, and Pedraza 2017; Pedraza, Cruz Nichols, and LeBrón 2017). Although immigrant policies purportedly focus on noncitizens, in practice these policies spill over to affect families, social networks, and broader communities that experience growth through immigration, regardless of legal status (Cruz Nichols, LeBrón, and Pedraza 2018; LeBrón et al. 2018a; Lopez 2019).

The impact of 21st-century restrictive immigration and immigrant policies and discourse on Latina/o and immigrant communities has been documented (Kline 2019; LeBrón et al. 2018a; LeBrón et al. 2018c; Lopez 2019; Novak, Geronimus, and Martinez-Cardoso 2017). In 2012–2013, 97% of persons deported from the United States were of Latin American origin, and almost 70% were Mexican nationals (TRAC 2014). De jure and de facto immigration and immigrant policies and practices conflate race with legal status, shaping societal ideologies, norms, institutional policies toward Latina/o immigrants, and ultimately Latinas/os' experiences of interpersonal discrimination, stigma, and mistrust (Hatzenbuehler et al. 2017; Romero 2011). Immigration raids, increased discrimination, and concern about deportation are linked with adverse mental, birth, metabolic, and cardiovascular outcomes (LeBrón et al. 2018c; Novak, Geronimus, and Martinez-Cardoso 2017; Torres et al. 2018). Restrictive immigration and immigrant policies deteriorate health through pathways including policies and institutional and systems practices that restrict health-promoting opportunities, racialized stressors, barriers to accessing health-relevant resources (e.g., government-issued IDs, welfare benefits), and reduced health care access (Castañeda et al. 2015; LeBrón et al. 2018a; LeBrón et al., 2018b; LeBrón et al., 2019a; Wallace et al. 2019). To date, few studies (see, for example, Viruell-Fuentes 2007, 2011) have illuminated the health implications of how Latinas/os construct and negotiate their racialized identities amid the constraints of restrictive immigration and immigrant policies.

Racialization Processes and Policy Contexts

The scholarship on how Latinas/os form, contend with, and navigate their identities in the context of restrictive immigrant policies suggests that community-level and demographic variations may shape racialization processes and the strategies used to navigate those experiences. For example, Viruell-Fuentes and colleagues (2007) found that among Mexican-origin women living in a long-standing predominantly Latina/o neighborhood in a northern border community, relative to immigrant women, second-generation women recounted more frequent and painful experiences of discrimination and othering—a process of differentiating and stigmatizing a minoritized group (Grove and Zwi 2006; Viruell-Fuentes 2007). The authors theorized that second-generation women's activities outside their neighborhood and the cumulation of experiences with US institutions (e.g., schools) over the life course may shape their naming of and experiences with discrimination. More recently, Dreby (2013) found that when Latina/o children in an established Latina/o community experienced discrimination based on nativity, they deemphasized their place of birth or that of family members. In contrast, children in a town with a small Latina/o community who experienced race/ethnicity-based discrimination deemphasized their Mexican and Spanish-speaking backgrounds, regardless of their nativity. These findings suggest that processes of racialization and identity management strategies enacted may be shaped by the social context in which they unfold and by generational status.

Scholarship by LeBrón and colleagues (2018a) found that in their day-to-day interactions, Mexican-origin women navigated an intricate web of policies, institutions, and institutional agents in which authorities engaged multiple racializing markers or symbols of (il)legality to assess legal status. Driver's licenses were central racializing markers in these interactions, as were physical features (e.g., dark skin and hair), speaking Spanish or having an accent, being born outside the United States, and having an "ethnic" name. Based on assessments of legal status, institutional agents such as police, immigration officials, clerks who issue driver's licenses, and social welfare providers exercised authority over women and members of their networks within their jurisdiction, often circumscribing access to health-promoting resources. At issue is how women negotiated their identities within a context that continually assessed and stigmatized their multiple identities, including race/ethnicity, gender, nativity, class, and legal status. While the aforementioned study examined how institutions and institutional actors racialized Mexican-origin women, this study queries how women navigated their identities amid this dynamic context of racialization and their interactions with legal institutions, with implications for health processes.

A gap in this literature is the study of how Latinas engage agency in racialization processes and implications for health, particularly under the constraints of multiple restrictive immigration and immigrant policies. This study heeds the call by Wallace and De Trinidad Young (2018: 437) to "place the impact of [immigrant] policies in historical context—including the racialization of immigrant policy politics—and incorporate the agency of immigrants and advocates in policy advocacy." Understanding how Latinas/os navigate their identities amid restrictive immigrant policies as a form of agency and resistance to racialization may enhance understanding of variations in how these processes affect Latinas/os' everyday lives and the implications for health. Another gap is the study of health as a process, considering how immigration and immigrant policies and responses to racialization may accumulate and shape health over the life course.

Health Implications of Women's Experiences with Exclusionary Immigration and Immigrant Policies

The growing literature regarding the gendered and health implications of restrictive immigration and immigrant policies for Latinas has largely focused on implications for prenatal and perinatal health care utilization and birth outcomes (Novak, Geronimus, and Martinez-Cardoso 2017; Rhodes et al. 2015; Toomey et al. 2014), which are important consequences that affect health across multiple generations. Additionally, data indicate that men (85%) constitute the majority of deportations of persons of Latin American origin in the early 21st century (Golash-Boza and Hondagneu-Sotelo 2013). Less is known about how Mexican-origin women manage their racialized and gendered identities in a context that stigmatizes their identities or how these experiences and responses to racialization may shape health over the life course. With some exceptions (see, for example, Lopez 2019), few studies to date have explicitly examined how women from immigrant communities targeted by exclusionary immigration and immigrant policies contend with racialization processes linked with these policies and the implications for women's identities, health, and well-being over the life course.

Racialization and Immigrant Policies in Detroit

Reflecting ongoing race-based residential segregation in Detroit, Southwest Detroit is often dubbed "Mexicantown," highlighting race-based residential segregation and the long-standing and vibrant Latina/o community, many of whom are of Mexican origin (Data Driven Detroit 2013). Southwest Detroit is a largely low-income neighborhood along the US-Canada border, in a city that has experienced substantial economic disinvestment (Schulz et al. 2002; Sugrue 1996). An international bridge to Canada crosses through Southwest Detroit, rendering Southwest Detroit a site where enhanced interior and border immigration enforcement compound the surveillance of residents. Furthermore, in response to the REAL ID Act of 2005, in 2008 Michigan began denying access to driver's licenses and state-issued IDs for persons who could not prove their authorized US presence (Cox 2007).

In Detroit, low-income Mexican-origin residents have been found to have higher allostatic load—indicating stress-related dysregulation of multiple somatic systems—than Mexican-origin counterparts across the United States (Geronimus et al. 2020). One study found that from 2002 to 2008, immigrant Latinas/os in Detroit experienced greater increases in blood pressure linked with increased discrimination, relative to US-born Latinas/os (LeBrón et al. 2018c). This literature begins to illuminate the life course health impacts of multiple structural inequities for Latinas/os.

In this study, we examine how Mexican-origin women and their coethnics—members of the racial/ethnic group with which they identify—form, negotiate, and manage their racialized identities in a northern border community during a protracted period of restrictive immigrant policies (2013–2014), and within a context that blurs the boundaries between Latinas/os, immigrants, and unauthorized immigrants. This qualitative inquiry provides context to more fully understand the public health literature regarding racialization, restrictive immigration and immigrant policies, and health, through the lens of women's experiences. We address these questions using a grounded theory analysis of individual interviews with Mexican-origin women—themselves immigrants or children of immigrants—living in Southwest Detroit.

Methods

This study was born out of discussions with the Healthy Environments Partnership (HEP), a community-based participatory research partnership that has been working since 2000 to understand and address social inequities that shape cardiovascular inequities in Detroit (Schulz et al. 2005). Discussions of the heightened and pervasive system of immigrant policing in Southwest Detroit and implications for Latina/o residents' health and participation in physical activity were a crucial impetus for this study. The Detroit Hispanic Development Corporation (DHDC) is a founding and active member of HEP and has been serving the Latina/o community in Southwest Detroit and beyond since 1997. DHDC was a key partner in this study—shaping the research approach, guiding the data collection process, supporting recruitment, and interpreting and disseminating findings. To facilitate recruitment, we also collaborated with LA SED, a community-based organization (CBO) with two locations in Southwest Detroit.

Data Collection

Interviews were conducted from 2013 to 2014 with first- (n = 25), 1.5- (n = 10), and second-generation (n = 13) Mexican-origin women 18 years of age and older who lived in Southwest Detroit and were fluent in Spanish or English (table 1). Following Rumbaut (1994), *first generation* was defined as Mexico-born women who came to the United States when they were 12 years of age and older; *1.5 generation* includes Mexico-born women who came to the United States when they were younger than 12 years of age; and *second generation* comprises US-born women with one or both parents born in Mexico. The University of Michigan IRB approved this study in July 2013.

To recruit participants, the research team, including DHDC staff, identified community members who met the eligibility criteria and invited them to participate. The interviewers (AMWL, CG) shared information about the study at DHDC, and LA SED shared study information with clients who met the eligibility criteria. When speaking with clients directly and discussing the study with CBO staff, the research team described the study as an opportunity for eligible women to share their experiences with immigrant policies and to talk about their health. We noted that while the study may have limited benefits to participants, the findings had potential to inform recommendations for inclusive programs and policies to support immigrant communities. Following a snowball sampling approach (Patton

Table 1 Sociodemographic Characteristics of Study Participants: First, 1.5, and Second-Generation Mexican-Origin Women, Detroit, Michigan

	First generation (n = 25)		1.5 generation (n = 10)		Second generation (n = 13)	
	% (n)	Median (SD)	% (n)	Median (SD)	% (n)	Median (SD)
Age (years)		45.0 (11.3)		32.8 (14.5)		40.7 (19.0)
Interviewed in Spanish	96% (24)		40% (4)		23% (3)	
High school education or higher	48% (12)		80% (8)		69% (9)	
Employed in formal labor force	8% (2)		60% (6)		31% (4)	
Married or living with partner	96% (24)		50% (5)		38% (5)	
Live in household with 1+ child	88% (22)		70% (7)		77% (10)	
Self-rated fair or poor health	44% (11)		20% (2)		46% (6)	

1990), we asked participants and LA SED to share study information within their networks. Three quarters of participants were recruited through the networks of the study team and DHDC. The remaining one quarter were recruited through snowball sampling, facilitated by LA SED, and generally included women who identified as second generation and with more protected legal status. Interviews were completed at participants' homes or at one of the CBOs, according to participants' preferences.

Two authors (AMWL, CG) conducted semistructured individual interviews with participants. Both interviewers identified as Latina and are US citizens. The first author's identity as a Puerto Rican scholar and the third author's positionality as being of Mexican origin, personal experiences with immigrant policies, and connections to grassroots efforts in the local immigrant community may have facilitated connections with participants. We did not ask about legal status in an effort to safeguard participant information, but some participants chose to disclose their legal status or the status of someone they knew in the context of the interview. The interview guide was designed to include topics that could be addressed in an open-ended manner and in an order that was conducive to eliciting women's descriptions of their experiences. Discussion topics included experiences with immigration and immigrant policies, changes in immigrant policies and immigration enforcement practices, responses to immigrant policies and sentiments toward immigrants, experiences of discrimination, women's characterizations of their health, and recommendations for policy makers. During the verbal informed consent process, researchers asked the participants for permission to make an audio recording of the interview. At the end of interviews, women completed a brief closed-ended questionnaire. Participants received a $20 cash incentive and information about immigrant rights. In cases where particular needs arose, the research team provided information about relevant services.

Interviews ranged from one to three hours and were completed in participants' preferred language (Spanish: n = 31; English: n = 17). All audio-recorded interviews were transcribed verbatim. To protect participants, identifying information disclosed in the interview was not transcribed, and pseudonyms are used to refer to participants. The first author translated quotes from Spanish-language interviews.

Data Analysis

Following a grounded theory approach, we identified inductive themes by first applying an open coding scheme to initial interviews during data collection (Charmaz 2012; Corbin and Strauss 2008; Glaser and Strauss 1967). The research team discussed emerging findings throughout the data collection and analysis process. This facilitated the development of an emerging coding scheme and provided opportunities to engage in expert checking and reflect on the possible influence of the research process on the accounts that women shared. We organized segments of text into codes that were then grouped into categories and themes. This coding structure was applied to subsequent interviews and updated as new codes emerged. We used axial coding to identify connections across codes and categories and examined patterns within and across interviews to iteratively identify, interpret, and refine the inductive themes (Charmaz 2012; Glaser and Strauss 1967). Women frequently described not only their own experiences and actions but also those of other family members and friends (including their husbands and sons), illustrating how network members protect against the disclosure of legal status. In presenting the findings below we include descriptions of the experiences and actions of members of women's social networks as well as the personal experiences of the women who participated in the interviews.

Findings

Women's narratives suggest that institutional agents and peers (agents of racialization who were not representing a particular institution) often did not discern between an unauthorized legal status and noncitizen legal statuses (e.g., legal permanent resident, temporary protected status, U-visa holders). Accordingly, women often navigated a false binary of legal statuses: that of US citizen or unauthorized immigrant. We use the term "symbols of (il)legality" to describe commonly invoked racialized indicators of unauthorized legal status, often interpreted using the false binary described here. Our focus is on efforts described to subvert or disrupt those interpretive frames. The theme *resistance to the symbolic construction as an "other"* encompasses strategies that participants described using to subvert processes that contribute to the construction of racially minoritized groups. This theme included data from interviews in which women described strategies that they or their social network members used to respond to or resist racialization. It is characterized by three categories: constructing an authorized immigrant identity, engaging in immigration advocacy, and resisting stigmatizing labels (table 2). In presenting our findings below, we illustrate the dynamic and contingent nature of women's negotiation of multiple intersecting identities and statuses. In the following

Table 2 Resistance to the Symbolic Construction as an "Other" Grounded Theory: Categories and Subcategories

Theme: resistance to the symbolic construction of an "other"	
Category	Subcategory
1. Constructing an authorized immigrant identity	▪ Obscuring an unauthorized legal status ▪ Embracing an ascribed authorized immigrant identity
2. Engaging in immigration advocacy	
3. Resisting stigmatizing labels	

sections, we present both the categories that constitute this theme and our interpretation of findings and potential pathways by which these processes may shape health.

1. Constructing an Authorized Immigrant Identity

Women described multiple strategies to construct an authorized immigrant identity by distancing themselves from or concealing an unauthorized legal status. Subcategories encompassed efforts to obscure an unauthorized legal status and embrace an ascribed authorized immigrant identity.

Obscuring an Unauthorized Legal Status. Women in the 1.5 generation (regardless of legal status) described strategic actions that they, or members of their social networks, used to actively hide their unauthorized legal status from institutional officials, employers, and (often white) peers. Often, this approach involved using and/or concealing symbols such as their ethnic identity, reasons for not having a current driver's license, and ankle monitors, often interpreted as signs of (il)legality. In several cases, this approach involved constructing narratives for why individuals did not have state-issued identification. This strategy was invoked at work, in police encounters, and when non-Latino neighbors or other peers explicitly queried about legal status.

The construction of an authorized identity was one strategy used to avert the "gaze" (Foucault 1977) of (often white) peers that inquired about legal status. Susana, a 46-year-old first-generation woman, shared her concerns about a neighbor who she believed called immigration officials on another neighbor:

> So, he would ask my son, "Uh do you all have papers?" [My son said] "Yes, my father has papers and he is fixing it for my mother." He said,

> "Yes, he is from Los Angeles and he has his papers and everything." And he said, "And the woman that lives in front too?" [And my son said] "Yes, she is also American." He [neighbor] said, "Why . . . doesn't she speak English?" He noticed everything, that man. He [neighbor] said, "And why doesn't she speak English?" He [son] said, "Because she married a Mexican man and the Mexican [man] taught her to speak Spanish and she likes Spanish" [laugh]. . . . And he [son] would say to us, "Mama! If the man asks you if you have your papers, tell him yes, right?" He [son] said, "Tell him yes because he is asking me if [another neighbor] also has her papers." And I told him, "Yes, we all have them, also those over there and . . . everyone."

Susana's narrative illustrates a strategy intended to quell peers' questions about legal status. Notably, Susana's US-born son contributed to the construction of a protected identity for his family and neighbors, illustrating the engagement of women's social networks as part of collective efforts to resist racialization.

Women also described constructing an alternative identity in efforts to ward off adverse consequences. Angela, a 1.5-generation woman, described her husband's active construction of a different narrative at work:

> You know if you don't have a license, you don't get paid. . . . Like, he [husband] told his boss he doesn't have a license 'cause he has a DUI, which he doesn't [laughs], but, he had to lie. He said he doesn't have a license because he has a DUI and they didn't let him renew it, so, his boss tells him, like, he's not able to drive the trucks or nothin,' so he doesn't get paid as well as he should be, you know, because of the license.

This narrative provides a plausible explanation for not having a driver's license, thereby avoiding disclosure of unauthorized status. While the narrative also has costs, resulting in lower pay and restrictions on work activities, they are perhaps less severe than the consequences of revealing unauthorized legal status. Furthermore, claiming a DUI rather than disclosing an unauthorized legal status points to efforts to maintain dignity amid a societal and policy backdrop that racializes and criminalizes unauthorized legal status.

Women whose driver's licenses had expired described interactions with officials in which they obscured the reasons for their lack of a valid driver's license. As Angela explained:

> It's scary [laughs]. I've been pulled over once and, by a state police . . . and, well I lied to him, I told him that, that I was staying in Chicago for a couple of months so, when I—I barely had come back and I couldn't

> renew my license, and he just gave me a ticket for that and he told me, "As soon as you go renew it, you won't have to pay nothin' so just go renew it and"—and back then you . . . would be able to just pay the ticket off, but now, they're making you go to court for it.

Officials serve as gatekeepers for critical health-relevant resources (e.g., social welfare assistance, driver's license), and encounters with officials in which unauthorized legal status is disclosed can lead to severe consequences (e.g., detention, deportation). The driver's license was the most common symbol of (il)legality described in encounters with police and in interpersonal interactions with coethnics and white peers. Strategies to hide unauthorized status are crucial to mitigating policies that racially minoritize Mexican-origin women. Women and their network members attempted to *prevent* encounters where an official (e.g., police) could threaten to or contact immigration officials. Outcomes depended on other resources available to women such as English fluency.

Other women described managing their identities to prevent discrimination and loss of access to employment. Dalilia, a 1.5-generation single mother, was required to wear an ankle monitor upon release from immigration detention. She explained:

> I was working with fake papers. If they realize that when you see someone with one of those bands [ankle monitors] on you, what is the first thing you think? That this guy did something. They killed, stole, or something they have it that way. And well what was the owner [boss] going to think? Of me? I mean I didn't want to attract attention for them and, and I had it, I had like all loose pants that were ugly on me [laughter] and um, I hid it.

Dalilia concealed the ankle monitor to prevent attention and avoid having to disclose her legal status to the public, her coworkers, and her employer. This strategy was also imperative for maintaining her job, which she obtained by misleading employers about her legal status. Dalilia also managed her identity against the criminalizing message of the ankle monitor among peers, reflecting concern that she would be stigmatized. Later in the interview, she recalled reaching a point where she said "okay I'm going to decide to ignore" others' opinions about the ankle monitor. This decision was undertaken in nonwork contexts in which her identity felt safer (e.g., religious celebrations, when with close friends who are coethnics). This illustrates the ways that women weighed the costs and benefits of obscuring an unauthorized immigrant identity, and the ways in which these costs and benefits were contextual and situation-specific.

Embracing an Ascribed Authorized Immigrant Identity. Women also described strategies that embrace an ascribed identity of having an authorized legal status, namely one ascribed by officials or peers. These actions often involved embracing ascribed racial/ethnic identities—and thus legal status, given the conflation of Mexican origin, nativity, and legal status—and assumptions made on the basis of having or not having a current driver's license. Immigrants leveraged this approach when working, when in the company of non-Latino peers, and when pursuing health and social services. Alicia, a 29-year old US citizen in the 1.5 generation whose dark-skinned husband was unauthorized until recently, explained his experience landscaping a US Border Patrol agent's house:

> [He] [d]oesn't look very Mexican. They didn't question it. And his name is . . . Arabic. Um, so when he introduced himself as [his name], he just says [husband's first name, name of company husband works for]. So, when I've talked to other people who are lighter skinned or who have resembled more Mexican features or on their trucks have the [Mexican] flag, or something, the stories that they tell me and the things that they share is that they have been more racially profiled. [They say] . . . "They looked at me, they pulled me over intentionally." My brother-in-law . . . looks very Hispanic, [like a] cowboy. He was like pulled over three different times on the same [emphasis] road, by the same [emphasis] cop. . . . I wonder if that has to do with how they are racially profiling people.

Alicia's account illustrates how peers invoke skin color and occupation as symbols of (il)legality. These socially constructed symbols also intersect with geography (i.e., residence near a large Arab American community). Generally, women perceived Arab Americans as subject to less immigrant-policing-related surveillance, and a few women described protections incurred by being classified as Arab American. Symbols included the racial background ascribed to their name and/or ambiguous physical features. However, generally women identified looking Arabic as protective for men, but not for women. The discussion section addresses this perceived gendered protective function of ascribed Arab identities, in a context in which Arab Americans have experienced high levels of anti-Arabic sentiments (Lauderdale 2006).

Rebecca, a 41-year-old first-generation woman, had a valid driver's license, which led to assumptions regarding her eligibility to vote. When those assumptions came into play at a local community health center, she did not challenge them:

> Well, when I show them my ID they think I have papers and they ask, "Are you going to vote for . . . ?" . . . I tell them no, but they don't ask me why, they just think that I have the right to vote.

In her interview Rebecca identified numerous social agents who equated a driver's license with US citizenship, including social welfare caseworkers and staff at a local community health center. In these situations, she routinely did not contest an assumed citizenship status, preventing questions about her legal status and the restriction of access to health care and social services. Consistent with the strategy of obscuring symbols of (il)legality, women managed their identities in the context of local "get out the vote" organizing efforts.

These strategies illustrate women's and men's efforts to prevent disclosure of unauthorized legal status by manipulating the very symbols of (il)legality (e.g., nativity, driver's license, physical features) used by agents of racialization. The relative success of obscuring an unauthorized legal status often varied by, for example, access to resources such as a valid driver's license, language use, physical characteristics, names, and demographic contexts. Specifically, women in the first and 1.5 generations who were unauthorized generally described engaging in these strategies. Immigrant women with an authorized legal status (e.g., citizen, resident, Deferred Action for Childhood Arrivals [DACA]) and those in the second generation with unauthorized immigrant family members likewise recalled family members engaging in these strategies as well as their own efforts to support these identity construction and management efforts.

Efforts to resist the symbolic construction as an "other" were continually engaged to resist or ameliorate stigmatizing perceptions of Mexican immigrants and immigration enforcement efforts that constructed their statuses and identities as an inferior "other." These strategies were also used to deflect encounters with individuals who they anticipated would construct them as different and consequently reinforce racialization. These strategies were ones that women chronically *anticipated* having to engage, reflecting women's attentiveness to and vigilance against the possibilities of encountering immigration officials, losing opportunities to work or receive services, or experiencing interpersonal discrimination. Thus, strategies such as obscuring a stigmatized identity were used to alleviate adverse consequences of racialization.

There are a number of important pathways through which strategic actions to hide an unauthorized immigrant identity may have health implications. Identity management processes (Goffman 1963) that seek to maintain access to social and material resources linked to legal status can protect against unemployment and encounters with immigration enforcement. However, chronic and effortful construction of an alternative identity requires substantial psychosocial resources. Over time, exposures to stressful political and social contexts and the identity management strategies required to navigate them may contribute to the deterioration of mental health (Pearlin et al. 1981). In the longer term, physical costs of such efforts may include risk of cardiovascular and metabolic conditions linked to stress over the life course (Geronimus et al. 2020; Jackson, Knight, and Rafferty 2010).

2. Engaging in Immigration Advocacy

The category *engaging in immigration advocacy* includes action such as participating in immigration policy advocacy or deportation deferral marches or protests, or signing petitions regarding immigration enforcement practices or policies or the release of persons in immigrant detention. Among women who described engaging in immigration advocacy, the catalyst was often a coethnic's immigrant detention or the opening of a window of opportunity to shape inclusive immigration and immigrant policies. Sometimes, immigration advocacy was in support of members of women's social networks and/or broader community. Most commonly, this category emerged in interviews with women in the 1.5 and second generations. Several women reported engaging in this strategy on behalf of someone who had been deported or was vulnerable to deportation; others reported advocating for the broader Latina/o community in Southwest Detroit.

Targeted advocacy efforts emerged when women knew or knew of an individual facing deportation. Alicia, a 29-year-old woman, is a US citizen and has lived in the US since she was an infant. Her husband was an unauthorized immigrant until recently. She explained her response to witnessing a parent's arrest by immigration officials outside her child's school:

> [A] parent was followed [by immigration officials] to my child's middle school. I didn't know the parent, but just seeing all of that happen, I was emotional. So it made my son emotional. So he's like, "I don't know why I'm crying." I'm like, "I don't know why I'm crying too. But it's just emotional. That's somebody's dad. That's somebody's husband. That could have been your dad." So it's just really emotional. And it affected

me in the entire day at work even though, um, I tend to leave home at home when I'm at work, but because that happened right in the transition of coming to work, I was kind of like, just . . . just distraught from the situation. Um, I don't know who the man was, but when they went to go advocate for him downtown—um, at the immigration, I went.

Alicia resonated with the experience through her witness of the arrest and her husband's own legal status, which was unauthorized until recently. Her emotional ties to her coethnics' experience contributed to her decision to participate in advocacy efforts to petition for the release of the student's father.

Fewer immigrant women who had an unauthorized legal status described engaging in immigration advocacy. For example, Rocio, a 36-year-old woman in the first generation who is an unauthorized immigrant, recalled, "Would you believe we went to Washington . . . like two years ago we went there for the marches . . . immigration." It is noteworthy that Rocio described participating in a national march hundreds of miles from Michigan, given her limited mobility because of restrictions on her ability to drive without a current driver's license. Rocio's participation may be understood in the context of her legal status. Her hope that she and her family might benefit from policy decisions related to advocacy efforts were reflected in her interview when she said, "I hope that when my son turns 21 that he can [change his legal status]."

Engaging in immigration advocacy may offer a way for women to connect to their community or identity in a *healing* manner, as opposed to strategies that seek to conceal their identity (Whyte 2014). This strategy may also offer a concrete way to support and advocate for themselves and/or coethnics (Cruz Nichols and Garibaldo Valdéz 2020). Thus, this strategy may reaffirm individual and collective identities vis-à-vis immigration and immigrant policies that racialize them and their coethnics and provide an opportunity to disrupt these processes.

Additionally, research indicates potential health benefits of some forms of political participation. Studies have linked political participation or activism with improved mental health outcomes for racially minoritized college students (Hope et al. 2018) and Black city council representation with favorable birth outcomes (LaVeist 1992). One study suggests that the salubrious benefits of political activism vary by form of activism (Klar and Kassner 2009). This literature theorizes that political participation may reflect strong community-level social organization; build sense of community, psychological empowerment, and/or community empowerment; and/or interrupt the pathways between racialized stressors such as discrimination and stress responses, anxiety, and depressive symptoms (Hope et al. 2018; LaVeist 1992; Wallerstein 1992). However, this literature also hypothesizes that for some, political activism could be linked with increases in discrimination that could be health deteriorating (Hope et al. 2018).

3. Resisting Stigmatizing Labels

The category *resisting stigmatized labels* includes efforts to resist labels that construct women and their network members as racially minoritized and that promulgate processes of racialization. For example, several women distanced themselves from the label "Mexican American," emphasizing they are "Mexican" and not "American." As Isabella, a woman in the second generation, explained:

> Whether you're born or not born in the United States, everybody has their own rights. . . . I mean what, I was born in Chicago, I was born here but I'm not American. Both of my parents are Mexican. There is no American blood in me. I am Mexican. I mean just because they say I was born here, I am Mexican American? Just because I was born here, okay, I get it, I was born here. What about it? None of their blood is in me, none of their cultures are in me. What my cultures—the way I celebrate Christmas, the way I celebrate, it's not how Americans celebrate. I celebrate how Mexicans celebrate it. All my culture, all of that, it's more Mexican than anything.

Here, Isabella grapples with the dissonance between her birthright citizenship and her family's social and economic exclusion, which manifest through constrained mobility, policing, detention, and deportation of her loved ones. She recognizes that her US citizenship does not afford her the same privileges of other US citizens. This reference to non-Latino whites as "Americans" may indicate women's resistance to classifying themselves with this national identity in a country that they feel largely excludes them, instead they embrace identities such as their ethnic identity and/or national origin or descent. Embracing their non-American identity also illustrates how women worked to construct and maintain an affirming Mexican identity in response to a context that stigmatizes their Mexican heritage. As with Isabella, several women in the 1.5 and second generations emphasized that there is no "American" heritage in them. These statements were less common among first-generation women.

This approach may be understood as a way of asserting a self that resists stigmatizing labels attached to Mexican American identity. Emphatic distancing from terms that may suggest superficial assimilation in the United States, such as "Mexican American," may reflect responses to experiences that racialize women as not belonging in the United States or as Americans. The health implications of this strategy of resistance may vary according to the typologies of racialization experienced. For example, earlier in the interview Isabella shared multiple consequences of immigration enforcement in her life: her mother's deportation, the separation of her family, and the imprisonment of her brothers. Her experiences may contribute to active construction of an identity that resists labels ascribed by institutions and individuals that create and reinforce the stigmatization of Mexican-origin peoples. Similarly, Viruell-Fuentes and Schulz (2011) reported a similar embracing of Mexican culture and identity among second-generation Mexican-origin women, while distancing from an identity as "American."

Women also engaged in direct acts of resistance to racialized stereotypes, while simultaneously asserting a valued identity as Mexican. Alice, a 50-year-old second-generation woman, explained the tensions between affirming her ethnic identity and resisting racialized stereotypes when encountering police in her neighborhood during a traffic stop:

> One time I was stopped by the police . . . and um the police as they are walking up on me . . . the police officer tells the police officer, "Uh, it's another one of those that doesn't know how to speak English." And then when she got to the [car] door I said, "Yes, I do know how to speak English, I speak English." And I think it's all because of the way I look. I look real Mexican, and people ask for my documentation. Basically, I'm always like in a hoodie, so I get that look, you know. I think it has to do with my appearance. The way I dress, the way I carry myself, but—I speak Spanish when I can, you know, with my kids and stuff, when . . . I listen to Mexican music, so people probably just assume that I don't know English.

As Alice implied, her efforts to assert and affirm her identity in her everyday life also heighten her risk of encounters with immigrant policing systems. Her account also illustrates how this active form of resistance is contingent on resources. Alice, who was born in the United States and is bilingual, possessed the linguistic skills to demonstrate her authorized legal status when visibly asserting her identity. Alternatively, for first-generation women, those who were primarily Spanish speakers, and those who were unauthorized immigrants, the risks associated with direct resistance to racialized stereotypes may have been much greater.

Legal Status, Situational Context, and Resistance to the Symbolic Construction as an "Other." These identities that women and members of their social networks actively managed provided a diverse set of malleable resources on which they could draw in responding to racialization. Their narratives suggest agency is itself shaped by the social structures in which they are embedded. Women and members of their networks who were unauthorized immigrants had access to a limited range of resources—including the same symbols of (il)legality and network members who could participate in these actions—to draw on when responding to racialization. The success of their efforts to negotiate these identities have implications for the preservation of work opportunities, access to health and social services, and preventing detention, deportation, and family separation. Women who had an unauthorized legal status or who had unauthorized network members generally reported greater effects of racialization on their lives than those with authorized legal statuses and described more constrained access to resources to resist the use of racializing markers in their day-to-day lives.

Discussion

Above, we describe themes that emerged from our analysis of Mexican-origin women's responses to racialization processes that unfolded during a period of increasingly restrictive immigration and immigrant policies and policing. Strategies varied according to the situational context and the resources women and other members of their social networks had available. Based on interpretation of the findings described above, the health implications of responses to processes of racialization may also intersect with other responses to affect health in the short and long term. Women's accounts illustrate the dynamic nature of socially structured opportunities and challenges and demonstrate their agency in actively managing identities and constructions within those contexts.

Health Implications of Resisting Symbolic Construction as an "Other"

Women negotiated racialization processes in part by resisting the construction of themselves as "other." They did so by leveraging the very symbols of (il)legality used by officials and peers. For example, women used the driver's license—a key racializing marker and symbol of legal status—to shield themselves and network members from scrutiny about legal status and protect themselves against threats to health and social, economic, and political well-being. Additionally, some women transposed symbols of (il)legality such as their Mexican origin by asserting an affirming Mexican identity. Such actions countered the stigmatizing identities constructed by white-dominant social institutions and perpetuated by cultural racism, which often cast Mexican-origin communities as threats and undeserving, and therefore exploitable (LeBrón et al. 2018a). The health implications of these strategies are likely contingent on experiences with racialization processes, the resources on which women and their network members can draw, and other responses to racialization. Furthermore, some strategies may protect health in the short term but have health-threatening potentials in the intermediate and longer term. For example, efforts to hide an unauthorized immigrant identity may prevent immigrant detention and deportation, thus preserving access to social, economic, and material resources while also taking a toll on mental well-being. Over the longer term, prolonged engagement of strategies to prevent confrontations with the immigrant policing infrastructure may exact health consequences through the dysregulation of multiple biological systems (Geronimus et al. 2020). How these health consequences unfold may depend on contextual factors and individual and network resources (Geronimus et al. 2020; LeBrón et al. 2019b). We now consider and discuss mechanisms by which these processes may affect health.

Our findings suggest that particularly 1.5- and second-generation women asserted their Mexican identities, affirmed Mexican cultural practices, and preserved Spanish language use despite institutional officials using these factors as racializing markers. These forms of resistance emerged to subvert racial stigmatization and associated mistreatment (Sánchez Gibau 2005). One strategy to resist being symbolically constructed as "other" included constructing a valued social identity. Goffman (1963: 14) notes that a stigmatized individual is "likely to feel that [s]he is 'on,' having to be self-conscious and calculating about the impression [s]he is making, to a degree and in areas of conduct which [s]he assumes others are not." Thus, careful strategies to manage discreditable identities may be consequences of occupying a vulnerable place in a social hierarchy. While immigration and immigrant policies and associated ideologies racialized Mexican-origin women as inferior in the US racial classifications system, they actively worked to distinguish, preserve, and emphasize their Mexican identities. The stress process framework (Pearlin et al. 1981) suggests that these identity management processes may shape access to political resources, economic resources, social support, and health care, all of which can shape health and render these negotiations matters of life, death, longevity, deportation, and/or family separation. Moreover, active and effortful practices to construct or preserve identities vis-à-vis racial classification systems may be a chronic response that poses longer-term health risks. For example, the John Henryism hypothesis (James 1994) suggests that the exertion of significant psychosocial resources to manage devalued identities may contribute to physiological dysregulation.

Engaging in immigration advocacy to resist processes of racialization may have multiple health-relevant implications. It may help to protect community members from deportation and/or mobilize social support in that process. It may impact policy decisions with implications for immigrant well-being. It is also possible that engaging in immigration advocacy can serve to enhance or activate social networks that are potential sources of emotional and instrumental social support. This form of resistance may operate to affirm women's identities in a context in which they are stigmatized. Additionally, participating in immigration advocacy may facilitate resistance of ascribed and stigmatized identities, offering positive and empowered identities as alternatives. Engaging in immigration advocacy may simultaneously expose women and/or their network members to stressors that derive from increased visibility and may enhance their risk for immigration enforcement.

Resisting labels and content associated with stigmatized identities also has complex implications for health. For example, women described efforts to construct and validate an affirming ethnic identity vis-à-vis the "American" identities from which they recognize they are largely excluded. In a heightened context of nativism and xenophobia, this strategy may offer a form of resistance to anti-immigrant racialization processes (Omi and Winant 2015). Thus, women's sense of belonging or not belonging and their use of the term "American" to refer to non-Latino whites may reflect their experiences of and resistance to racialization and the contexts in which women are located. For example, several unauthorized immigrant women perceived strategies to exercise and affirm their identity as increasing their risk for othering from police or immigration officials. In contrast, women with more protected legal statuses tended to describe explicit strategies to exercise their identity in relation to the immigration enforcement infrastructure, either in direct encounters with institutional officials or through immigration advocacy. Thus, both the ability to engage this strategy and its health implications may depend on the resources women can use to prevent or resist racialization processes. These resources are shaped by social position, including but not limited to legal status.

Future Research

These findings illuminate several areas for future research. First, because women's experiences with and responses to racialization were contingent on their vulnerabilities to and protections from these processes, future studies should examine variations in experiences of and responses to racialization across and within Latina/o subgroups. Second, future research might empirically test hypotheses about the experiences of and dynamics between multiple racial/ethnic groups with immigration and immigrant policies, sentiments, and practices, and the implications for health, including the potentially gendered nature of these dynamics. For example, several women in this study perceived that Arab Americans in the Detroit area were less vulnerable to racialization than Latinas/os. In particular, participants described instances when male, but not female, coethnics who were racialized as Arab American averted interactions with immigration officials. It is plausible that these processes are gendered with, for example, Arab American and Latina women being more distinguishable through different forms of dress (e.g., hijab) or that indicators of Arab or Latino race engaged in racialization processes for men may be subtler and only apparent after closer interaction (e.g., a conversation). Other research indicates high levels of racial profiling and anti-Arab sentiments, particularly since 9/11 (Padela and Heisler 2010) and the 2016 change in presidential administrations (Lajevardi 2020), with these experiences associated with adverse health outcomes for Arab Americans (Lauderdale 2006; Padela and Heisler 2010). Thus, the perception that Arab Americans occupied a more protected social position than Latinas/os warrants further investigation. Third, studies are needed that explore gender differences in experiences of legal status inquiries and strategies to manage racialized identities. Such studies might explore gender differences in the frequency with and conditions in which legal status surfaces and the resources that are leveraged to respond to racializing encounters.

Strengths and Limitations

This study has several limitations. First, these findings are based on the narratives of a sample of Mexican-origin women in a largely low- to moderate-income neighborhood along the US-Canada border (Schulz et al. 2002) and during a period of changing immigrant policies (e.g., DACA, driver's license). The immigrant and social policy landscape continuously changes. These findings should be understood within the time period of this inquiry, this community, and an increasingly restrictive immigrant policy environment (2013–2014). Moreover, this study examined the experiences of Mexican-origin women, the largest subgroup of Latinas/os in the United States. Future research is necessary to examine these experiences with greater depth with other Latina/o subgroups.

Second, the racialization processes discussed are relational and dynamic. They intersect with gender, socioeconomic position, immigrant generation, legal status, and other social locations as well as linguistic and physical characteristics of involved individuals. This study discusses the gendered nature of these experiences through the perspectives of women, and it does not include an analysis based on men's descriptions. Garcia (2017), studying Mexican-origin women's experiences with anti-immigrant sentiments in 2009–2013 in Texas, described how women were racialized by institutional actors (i.e., police, health care providers) as hyperfertile and hypersexual. The findings presented here build upon scholarship that indicates the consequences of Mexican-origin women's experiences with immigration policies and sentiments and that illuminates women's agentic responses to racialization processes. Research into the experience and health of men is needed, including the social statuses that may affect them.

Third, this study of women's experiences with restrictive immigrant policies does not include the perspectives of "implicated actors" (Clarke and Montini 1993) or key individuals or social groups implicated for their role in racializing Mexican-origin women, such as immigration officials, police, clerks who issue driver's licenses, social and health care service providers, men, or children. Ethnographic studies (Kline 2019; Lopez 2019) provide additional insights into how agents of racialization contribute to Mexican-origin women's experiences with racism and xenophobia.

Strengths of this study include the focus on women's responses to racialization, enriching a literature that has largely focused unidirectionally on the impact of immigrant policies on Latina/o communities but has not fully examined feedback loops (Castañeda et al. 2015). Additionally, this study contributes an intersectional analysis of the interplay of multiple social statuses (e.g., legal status, language use) in negotiating racialized identities. Notably, while studies of the health implications of restrictive immigrant policies often focus on the American Southwest, new settlement communities, and states that have passed multiple restrictive immigrant policies, this case study sheds light on the experiences of women in a northern border community with an established Latina/o community.

Implications for Policy and Practice

These findings suggest several opportunities for intervention. First, this analysis highlights health implications of current policies that restrict access to political, economic, and social resources among those whose legal status is questioned. These policies and their health implications have impacts beyond those who are directly affected, with substantial social costs (Cruz Nichols, LeBrón, and Pedraza 2018; Pedraza, Cruz Nichols, and LeBrón 2017). Providing clear pathways to citizenship and other policies (e.g., driver's license, employment, welfare) that promote the full integration of Latina/o immigrants into US society are important tools with which to disrupt these currently costly dynamics (De Trinidad Young and Wallace 2021). For example, the temporary protected status provided to DACA recipients who migrated to the United States as young children has been linked with reduced stress and anxiety and improved cardiovascular and mental health, which could alleviate the social and economic burden of mental and cardiovascular health on the population (Giuntella and Lonsky 2020). Given the salience of legal status in women's daily lives, passage of immigration reform legislation that offers a clear pathway to citizenship holds strong potential for substantially improving health equity. Additionally, at the federal level, the American Public Health Association has called for the US presidential administration to enact inclusive immigrant policies, such as ensuring access to housing subsidies and other public benefits regardless of legal status, and to avoid linking use of public benefits with appeals for legalization (Benjamin 2019a, 2019b, 2021).

Second, a focus on inclusive state- and community-level policies can promote health and health equity. For example, providing access to driver's licenses for unauthorized immigrants may disrupt racialization and enhance access to social and economic resources. Policy and programmatic interventions (e.g., accepting a range of identifying documents for access to social and economic resources) that consider the health implications of racialization processes are urgently needed. Such changes hold potential for promoting the health of immigrant and US-born Latinas/os by alleviating stressful life contexts, affirming identities that have been persistently stigmatized, and improving access to health-promoting resources (LeBrón et al. 2019a; De Trinidad Young and Wallace 2021).

Conclusions

Findings from this study demonstrate the importance of social, political, and geographic contexts for the racialized forces acting on populations that experience health inequities. Furthermore, they describe Mexican-origin women's strategic actions to navigate those processes, highlighting the dynamic, negotiated, and contingent nature of those actions. Public health interventions to reduce health inequities in communities affected by restrictive immigration and immigrant policies would benefit from contextualizing Latinas/os' experiences of and responses to racialization as complex, dynamic, and agentic. They amplify the public health implications of national immigration and immigrant policy and the importance of supporting communities that are experiencing—and resisting—racialization as central to the promotion of health equity as a national priority.

■ ■ ■

Alana M. W. LeBrón is an assistant professor of health, society, and behavior and Chicano/Latino studies at the University of California, Irvine. Her scholarship focuses on mechanisms by which structural racism shapes the health of communities of color, with a focus on policies, systems, and environments. Much of her scholarship involves community-based participatory research, working in partnership with members of affected communities to strengthen understanding of the ways in which structural racism shapes health inequities and to develop and evaluate strategies that advocate for structural change, mitigate the health impacts of structural racism, and create new systems for promoting health equity.
alebron@uci.edu

Amy J. Schulz is a University Diversity and Social Transformation Professor of health behavior and health education at the University of Michigan School of Public Health. Her research focuses on social and physical environmental factors and their effects on health, health equity, and urban health. Much of her research is conducted with partners in Detroit through the Healthy Environments Partnership, which uses a community-based participatory research approach for understanding and addressing drivers of excess cardiovascular risk, conducting health impact assessments of proposed policies, and developing public health action plans for reducing air pollution and promoting health in Detroit and surrounding areas.

Cindy Gamboa is the community organizing and advocacy director at the Detroit Hispanic Development Corporation. Previously, she was the community coordinator for the Healthy Environments Partnership, a long-standing community-based participatory research partnership working to understand and address excess cardiovascular risk in Detroit. She also was active in several collaborations, programs, and policy-change initiatives for promoting health equity.

Angela Reyes is the executive director and founder of the Detroit Hispanic Development Corporation. She has expertise in critical policy issues that affect residents of Southwest Detroit and other urban areas, including positive youth development, youth violence, substance abuse, immigration, educational reform, community organizing, and community-based participatory research. She is a founding and active member of the Healthy Environments Partnership.

Edna Viruell-Fuentes was a professor of Latina/o studies at University of Illinois Urbana-Champaign. Her research focused on Latina/o and immigrant health; transnational processes, practices, and methods; and structural determinants of health contexts, including neighborhoods and immigration policies.

Barbara A. Israel is a professor of health behavior and health education at the University of Michigan School of Public Health. She has published widely in the areas of social and physical environmental determinants of health and health inequities; the relationship among stress, social support, and physical and mental health; and community-based participatory research. Since 1995, she has worked with academic and community partners to establish and maintain the Detroit Community-Academic Urban Research Center, which works to foster and support the development of equitable community-academic partnerships focused on understanding and addressing health inequities in Detroit.

Acknowledgments

We express our gratitude to the courageous women who warmly opened their hearts to share their experiences, steady perseverance, and hopes. We also acknowledge and graciously thank the late Edna Viruell-Fuentes for her contributions, including her rich theorization and surgical attention to research methods, which strengthened our theorization of the complex interplay of race, racism, and health; the research process; and the interpretation of findings. We hope this work honors her dedication to enriching the study of how structural racism shapes health processes for Latina/o communities. Thanks to the Detroit Hispanic Development Corporation, LA SED, James S. House, the Healthy Environments Partnership, Detroit Community-Academic Urban Research Center, Cristina Bernal, Kirsten Herold, William D. Lopez, Jessica Yen, and members of the Coalition for Interdisciplinary Research on Latina/o Issues at the University of Michigan for their comments on earlier versions of this work. Short excerpts from LeBrón and colleagues (2018) are republished here with permission from Springer

Nature. This research was supported by the Center for Research on Ethnicity, Culture, and Health; Rackham Graduate School; the Transportation Research Institute; the Center for the Education of Women; the Institute for Research on Women and Gender; the National Center for Institutional Diversity at the University of Michigan; and the National Institute of General Medical Sciences (R-25–058641). The results presented here are solely the responsibility of the authors and do not represent the views of the funders or the authors' employers.

References

Benjamin, Georges C. 2019a. "APHA Condemns the Administration's Finalized 'Public Charge' Rule." American Public Health Association, August 15. www.apha.org/News-and-Media/News-Releases/APHA-News-Releases/2019/Public-charge-rule.

Benjamin, Georges C. 2019b. Letter to the Department of Housing and Urban Development re: HUD Docket No. FR-6124-P-01, RIN 2501-AD89 Comments in Response to Proposed Rulemaking: Housing and Community Development Act of 1980: Verification of Eligible Status. American Public Health Association, July 3. www.apha.org/-/media/Files/PDF/advocacy/TestimonyAndComments/190703_APHA_Comments_HUD_Mixed_Status_Rule.ashx.

Benjamin, Georges C. 2021. "APHA Applauds President Biden's Executive Actions to Reunify Families and Provide Health Care to Legal Immigrants." American Public Health Association, February 2. www.apha.org/news-and-media/news-releases/apha-news-releases/2021/reunification.

Castañeda, Heide, Seth M. Holmes, Daniel S. Madrigal, Maria Elena De Trinidad Young, Naomi Beyeler, and James Quesada. 2015. "Immigration as a Social Determinant of Health." *Annual Review of Public Health* 36: 375–92. doi.org/10.1146/annurev-publhealth-032013–182419.

Charmaz, Kathy. 2012. "The Power and Potential of Grounded Theory." *Medical Sociology Online* 6, no. 3: 2–15. www.medicalsociologyonline.org/resources/Vol6Iss3/MSo-600x_The-Power-and-Potential-Grounded-Theory_Charmaz.pdf.

Chavez, Leo. 2013. *The Latino Threat: Constructing Immigrants, Citizens, and the Nation*. Stanford, CA: Stanford University.

Clarke, Adele, and Theresa Montini. 1993. "The Many Faces of RU486: Tales of Situated Knowledges and Technological Contestations." *Science, Technology, and Human Values* 18, no. 1: 42–78.

Coleman, Matthew, and Angela Stuesse. 2014. "Policing Borders, Policing Bodies: The Territorial and Biopolitical Roots of US Immigration Control." In *Placing the Border in Everyday Life*, edited by Reece Jones and Corey Johnson, 33–63. Burlington, VT: Ashgate Publishing Company.

Corbin, Juliet, and Anselm Strauss. 2008. *Basics of Qualitative Research*. 3rd ed. Thousand Oaks, CA: Sage Publications.

Cox, Mike. 2007. "Permanent Residency Requirement for Driver's Licenses, Opinion No. 7210." State of Michigan Attorney General, December 27. www.ag.state.mi.us/opinion/datafiles/2000s/op10286.htm.

Cruz Nichols, Vanessa, and Ramón Garibaldo Valdéz. 2020. "How to Sound the Alarms: Untangling Racialized Threat in Latinx Mobilization." *PS: Political Science and Politics* 53, no. 4: 690–96. doi.org/10.1017/S1049096520000530.

Cruz Nichols, Vanessa, Alana M. W. LeBrón, and Francisco I. Pedraza. 2017. "Policy Feedback: Government Skepticism Trickling from Immigration to Matters of Health." In *Policing and Race: Economic, Political, and Social Dynamics*, edited by James D. Ward, 85–108. Lanham, MD: Lexington Books.

Cruz Nichols, Vanessa, Alana M. W. LeBrón, and Francisco I. Pedraza. 2018. "Policing Us Sick: The Health of Latinos in an Era of Heightened Deportations and Racialized Policing." *Politics Symposium* 51, no. 2: 293–97.

Data Driven Detroit. 2013. "Southwest Detroit Neighborhoods Profile." July. datadrivendetroit.org/files/SGN/SW_Detroit_Neighborhoods_Profile_2013_081913.pdf.

De Genova, Nicholas. 2007. "The Production of Culprits: From Deportability to Detainability in the Aftermath of 'Homeland Security.'" *Citizenship Studies* 11, no. 5: 421–48. doi.org/10.1080/13621020701605735.

De Trinidad Young, Maria-Elena, and Steven P. Wallace. 2021. "A Window of Opportunity Is Opening to Improve Immigrant Health: A Research and Practice Agenda." *American Journal of Public Health* 111, no. 3: 398–401. doi.org/10.2105/ajph.2020.306128.

Dreby, Joanna. 2013. "The Modern Deportation Regime and Mexican Families: The Indirect Consequences for Children in New Destination Communities." In *Constructing Immigrant "Illegality": Critiques, Experiences, and Responses*, edited by Cecilia Menjívar and Daniel Kanstroom, 181–202. New York: Cambridge University Press.

Ford, Chandra L., Derek M. Griffith, Marino A. Bruce, and Keone L. Gilbert. 2019. *Racism: Science and Tools for the Public Health Professional*. Washington, DC: American Public Health Association.

Foucault, Michel. 1977. *Discipline and Punish: The Birth of the Prison*. New York: Vintage Books.

Garcia, San Juanita. 2017. "Racializing 'Illegality': An Intersectional Approach to Understanding How Mexican-Origin Women Navigate an Anti-Immigrant Climate." *Sociology of Race and Ethnicity* 3, no. 4: 474–90.

Geronimus, Arline T., Jay A. Pearson, Erin Linnenbringer, Alexa K. Eisenberg, Carmen Stokes, Landon D. Hughes, and Amy J. Schulz. 2020. "Weathering in Detroit: Place, Race, Ethnicity, and Poverty as Conceptually Fluctuating Social Constructs Shaping Variation in Allostatic Load." *Milbank Quarterly* 98, no. 4: 1171–218. doi.org/10.1111/1468-0009.12484.

Giuntella, Osea, and Jakub Lonsky. 2020. "The Effects of DACA on Health Insurance, Access to Care, and Health Outcomes." *Journal of Health Economics* 72: 1–18. doi.org/10.1016/j.jhealeco.2020.102320.

Glaser, Barney G., and Anselm L. Strauss. 1967. *The Discovery of Grounded Theory: Strategies for Qualitative Research*. Chicago: Aldine Publishing.

Goffman, Erving. 1963. *Stigma: Notes on the Management of a Spoiled Identity*. New York: Simon and Schuster.

Golash-Boza, Tanya, and Pierrette Hondagneu-Sotelo. 2013. "Latino Immigrant Men and the Deportation Crisis: A Gendered Racial Removal Program." *Latino Studies* 11, no. 3: 271–92. doi.org/10.1057/lst.2013.14.

Grove, Natalie J., and Anthony B. Zwi. 2006. "Our Health and Theirs: Forced Migration, Othering, and Public Health." *Social Science and Medicine* 62, no. 8: 1931–42. doi.org/10.1016/j.socscimed.2005.08.061.

Hatzenbuehler, Mark L., Seth J. Prins, Morgan Flake, Morgan Philbin, M. Somjen Frazer, Daniel Hagen, and Jennifer Hirsch. 2017. "Immigration Policies and Mental Health Morbidity among Latinos: A State-Level Analysis." *Social Science and Medicine* 174: 169–78. doi.org/10.1016/j.socscimed.2016.11.040.

Hope, Elan C., Gabriel Velez, Carly Offidani-Bertrand, Micere Keels, and Myles I. Durkee. 2018. "Political Activism and Mental Health among Black and Latinx College Students." *Cultural Diversity and Ethnic Minority Psychology* 24, no. 1: 26–39.

Jackson, James S., Katherine M. Knight, and Jane A. Rafferty. 2010. "Race and Unhealthy Behaviors: Chronic Stress, the HPA Axis, and Physical and Mental Health Disparities over the Life Course." *American Journal of Public Health* 100, no. 5: 933–39. doi.org/10.2105/AJPH.2008.143446.

James, Sherman A. 1994. "John Henryism and the Health of African-Americans." *Culture, Medicine, and Psychiatry* 18, no. 2: 163–82. doi.org/10.1007/BF01379448.

Klar, Malte, and Tim Kassner. 2009. "Some Benefits of Being an Activist: Measuring Activism and Its Role in Psychological Well-Being." *Political Psychology* 30, no. 5: 755–77.

Kline, Nolan. 2019. *Pathogenic Policing: Immigration Enforcement and Health in the US South*. New Brunswick, NJ: Rutgers University Press.

Lajevardi, Nazita. 2020. *Outsiders at Home: The Politics of American Islamophobia*. Cambridge: Cambridge University Press.

Lauderdale, Diane S. 2006. "Birth Outcomes for Arabic-Named Women in California before and after September 11." *Demography* 43, no. 1: 185–201. doi.org/10.1353/dem.2006.0008.

LaVeist, Thomas A. 1992. "The Political Empowerment and Health Status of African-Americans: Mapping a New Territory." *American Journal of Sociology* 97, no. 4: 1080–95.

LeBrón, Alana M. W., Amy J. Schulz, Cindy Gamboa, Angela Reyes, Edna A. Viruell-Fuentes, and Barbara A. Israel. 2018a. "'They Are Clipping Our Wings': Health Implications of Restrictive Immigrant Policies for Mexican-Origin Women in a Northern Border Community." *Race and Social Problems* 10, no. 3: 174–92. doi.org/10.1007/s12552–018–9238–0.

LeBrón, Alana M. W., Amy J. Schulz, Graciela B. Mentz, Cindy Gamboa, and Angela Reyes. 2018b. "Antihypertensive Medication Use: Implications for Inequities in Cardiovascular Risk and Opportunities for Intervention." *Journal of Health Care for the Poor and Underserved* 29, no. 1: 192–201.

LeBrón, Alana M. W., Amy J. Schulz, Graciela B. Mentz, Angela Reyes, Cindy Gamboa, Barbara A. Israel, Edna A. Viruell-Fuentes, and James S. House. 2018c. "Impact of Change over Time in Self-Reported Discrimination on Blood Pressure: Implications for Inequities in Cardiovascular Risk for a Multi-Racial Urban Community." *Ethnicity and Health* 25, no. 3: 323–41. doi.org/10.1080/13557858.2018.1425378.

LeBrón, Alana M. W., Keta Cowan, William D. Lopez, Nicole L. Novak, Maria Ibarra-Frayre, and Jorge Delva. 2019a. "The Washtenaw ID Project: A Government-Issued ID Coalition Working Toward Social, Economic, and Racial Justice and Health Equity." *Health Education and Behavior* 46, suppl. 1: 53S–61S. doi.org/10.1177/1090198119864078.

LeBrón, Alana M. W., Amy J. Schulz, Graciela B. Mentz, Barbara A. Israel, and Carmen A. Stokes. 2019b. "Social Relationships, Neighbourhood Poverty, and Cumulative Biological Risk: Findings from a Multi-Racial US Urban Community." *Journal of Biosocial Science* 51, no. 6: 799–816. doi.org/10.1017/S002193201900004X.

LeBrón, Alana M. W., and Edna A. Viruell-Fuentes. 2020. "Racism and the Health of Latina/o Communities." In *"Is It Race or Racism?" State of the Evidence and Tools for the Public Health Professional*, edited by Chandra L. Ford, Derek M. Griffith, Marino A. Bruce, and Keon L. Gilbert, 413–28. Washington, DC: American Public Health Association Press.

Lopez, William D. 2019. *Separated: Family and Community in the Aftermath of an Immigration Raid.* Baltimore: Johns Hopkins University Press.

Miller, Todd. 2014. *Border Patrol Nation: Dispatches from the Front Lines of Homeland Security.* San Francisco: City Lights Books.

Ngai, Mae M. 2004. *Impossible Subjects: Illegal Aliens and the Making of Modern America.* Princeton, NJ: Princeton University Press.

Novak, Nicole L., Arline T. Geronimus, and Aresha M. Martinez-Cardoso. 2017. "Change in Birth Outcomes among Infants Born to Latina Mothers after a Major Immigration Raid." *International Journal of Epidemiology* 46, no. 3: 839–49. doi.org/10.1093/ije/dyw346.

Omi, Michael, and Howard Winant. 2015. *Racial Formation in the United States.* 3rd ed. New York: Routledge.

Padela, Aasim I., and Michele Heisler. 2010. "The Association of Perceived Abuse and Discrimination after September 11, 2001, with Psychological Distress, Level of Happiness, and Health Status among Arab Americans." *American Journal of Public Health* 100, no. 2: 284–91. doi.org/10.2105/AJPH.2009.164954.

Patton, Michael Quinn. 1990. *Qualitative Evaluation and Research Methods.* Thousand Oaks, CA: Sage Publications.

Pearlin, Leonard I., Elizabeth G. Menaghan, Morton A. Lieberman, and Joseph T. Mullan. 1981. "The Stress Process." *Journal of Health and Social Behavior* 22, no. 4: 337–56. doi.org/10.2307/2136676.

Pedraza, Francisco, Vanessa Cruz Nichols, and Alana M. W. LeBrón. 2017. "Cautious Citizenship: The Deterring Effect of Immigration Issue Salience on Health Care Use and Bureaucratic Interactions among Latino US Citizens." *Journal of Health Politics, Policy and Law* 42, no. 5: 925–60.

Rhodes, Scott D., Lilli Mann, Florence M. Simán, Eunyoung Song, Jorge Alonzo, Mario Downs, Emma Lawlor, et al. 2015. "The Impact of Local Immigration Enforcement Policies on the Health of Immigrant Hispanics/Latinos in the United States." *American Journal of Public Health* 105, no. 2: 329–37. doi.org/10.2105/AJPH.2014.302218.

Romero, Mary. 2011. "Keeping Citizenship Rights White: Arizona's Racial Profiling Practices in Immigration Law Enforcement." *Law Journal for Social Justice* 1, no. 1: 97–113.

Rumbaut, Rubén G. 1994. "The Crucible Within: Ethnic Identity, Self-Esteem, and Segmented Assimilation among Children of Immigrants." *International Migration Review* 28, no. 4: 748–94. doi.org/10.1177/019791839402800407.

Sánchez Gibau, Gina. 2005. "Contested Identities: Narratives of Race and Ethnicity in the Cape Verdean Diaspora." *Identities: Global Studies in Culture and Power* 12, no. 3: 405–38. doi.org/10.1080/10702890500203702.

Schulz, Amy J., Srimathi Kannan, J. Timothy Dvonch, Barbara A. Israel, Alex Allen, Sherman A. James, James S. House, and James Lepkowski. 2005. "Social and Physical Environments and Disparities in Risk for Cardiovascular Disease: The Healthy Environments Partnership Conceptual Model." *Environmental Health Perspectives* 113, no. 12: 1817–25. doi.org/10.1289/ehp.7913.

Schulz, Amy J., David R. Williams, Barbara A. Israel, and Lora Bex Lempert. 2002. "Racial and Spatial Relations as Fundamental Determinants of Health in Detroit." *Milbank Quarterly* 80, no. 4: 677–707. doi.org/10.1111/1468-0009.00028.

Schwalbe, Michael, Sandra Godwin, Daphne Holdern, Douglas Schrock, Shealy Thompson, Michele Wolkomir, and Daphne Holden. 2000. "Generic Processes in the Reproduction of Inequality: An Interactionist Analysis." *Social Forces* 72, no. 2: 419–52. doi.org/10.2307/2675505.

Sugrue, Thomas J. 1996. *The Origins of the Urban Crisis: Race and Inequality in Postwar Detroit.* Princeton, NJ: Princeton University Press.

Toomey, Russell B., Adriana J. Umaña-Taylor, David R. Williams, Elizabeth Harvey-Mendoza, Laudan B. Jahromi, and Kimberly A. Updegraff. 2014. "Impact of Arizona's SB 1070 Immigration Law on Utilization of Health Care and Public Assistance among Mexican-Origin Adolescent Mothers and Their Mother Figures." *American Journal of Public Health* 104, suppl. 1: S28–S34. doi.org/10.2105/AJPH.2013.301655.

Torres, Jacqueline M., Julianna Deardoff, Robert B. Gunier, Kim G. Harley, Abbey Alkon, Katherine Kogut, and Brenda Eskenazi. 2018. "Worry about Deportation and Cardiovascular Disease Risk Factors among Adult Women: The Center for the Health Assessment of Mothers and Children of Salinas Study." *Annals of Behavioral Medicine* 52, no. 2: 186–93.

TRAC (Transactional Records Access Clearinghouse) Immigration. 2014. "ICE Deportations: Gender, Age, and Country of Citizenship." April 9. trac.syr.edu/immigration/reports/350/.

Viruell-Fuentes, Edna A. 2007. "Beyond Acculturation: Immigration, Discrimination, and Health Research among Mexicans in the United States." *Social Science and Medicine* 65, no. 7: 1524–35. doi.org/10.1016/j.socscimed.2007.05.010.

Viruell-Fuentes, Edna A. 2011. "'It's a Lot of Work': Racialization Processes, Ethnic Identity Formations, and Their Health Implications." *Du Bois Review* 8, no. 1: 37–52. doi.org/10.1017/S1742058X11000117.

Viruell-Fuentes, Edna A., and Amy J. Schulz. 2011. "Toward a Dynamic Conceptualization of Social Ties and Context: Implications for Understanding Immigrant and Latino Health." *American Journal of Public Health* 99, no. 12: 2167–75.

Wallace, Steven P., and Maria-Elena De Trinidad Young. 2018. "Immigration vs. Immigrant: The Cycle of Anti-Immigrant Policies." *American Journal of Public Health* 108, no. 4: 436–37.

Wallace, Steven P., Maria-Elena De Trinidad Young, Michael A. Rodriguez, and Clair D. Brindis. 2019. "A Social Determinants of Health Framework Identifying State-Level Immigrant Policies and Their Influence on Health." *SSM—Population Health* 7: 100316. doi.org/10.1016/j.ssmph.2018.10.016.

Wallerstein, Nina. 1992. "Powerlessness, Empowerment, and Health: Implications for Health Promotion Programs." *American Journal of Health Promotion* 6, no. 3: 197–205.

Whyte, Kyle Powys. 2014. "Indigenous Women, Climate Change Impacts, and Collective Action." *Hypatia* 29, no. 3: 599–616. doi.org/10.1111/hypa.12089.

Printed and bound by CPI Group (UK) Ltd, Croydon, CR0 4YY

13/04/2025

14656470-0003